THE MANY FACES OF GRIEF

Stories of Love, Loss, and Hope
From a Hospital Chaplain

by

Maryann Miller

THE MANY FACES OF GRIEF
Copyright © 2021 by Maryann Miller

Published by MCM Enterprises

Edited by ALTO Editing Services

Cover Design by Dany Russell

Cover Photo from Getty Images

Formatted by The Book Khaleesi

PRINTED IN THE UNITED STATES OF AMERICA

10 9 8 7 6 5 4 3 2 1

CONTENTS

ACKNOWLEDGEMENTS

Thanks to ALTO Editing for going above and beyond in looking at new material I sent after the first edit. I'm like the artist to whom the master has to say, "Put the brush down. The painting is finished."

I have much appreciation for the talented graphic artist, Dany Russell, who also went above and beyond in designing the cover, making all the little changes from draft to draft until we had the final version.

Lastly, many thanks to Caleb Pirtle III for his generous support of other authors.

For all the people
who graced my life with their stories.

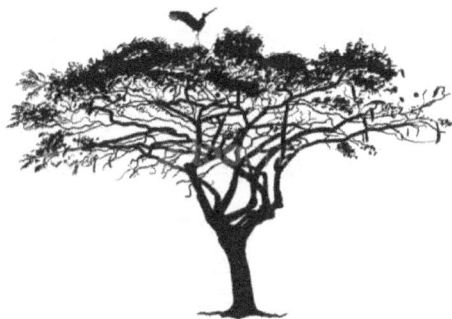

INTRODUCTION

"Peter, do you love me?"

"Master, you know I do."

"Then tend my sheep."

Those words are paraphrased from a Bible verse in John 21:15-17 where Jesus asks Simon Peter three times whether he loves Him. They are also words in a hymn that I sang frequently in choir. I loved the music, and the message in the lyrics stirred my heart to answer my baptismal call to discipleship. Maybe not the kind of discipleship that Peter and the others had so long ago, but something.

When my husband was ordained as a Permanent Deacon in the Roman Catholic Church, wives were invited, and encouraged, to "tend the sheep" in whatever way we could. I was already doing music ministry, which I loved, and my husband and I were in charge of the Family Life Program for the parish, but I never felt like that was quite enough.

1

THE MANY FACES OF GRIEF

About that same time, a good friend was in the hospital. I called her to see if she needed anything when I came to visit, and she said she'd love to receive Holy Communion. I'd never taken communion to somebody in the hospital before, but how hard could that be?

As it turned out, not hard at all. On the appointed day, my husband got a host from the tabernacle at church and brought it to me in a Pix, which is a special round container designed to hold consecrated hosts for communion. I went to the hospital armed with the Pix and my husband's prayer book, where he'd already pointed out where I could find the prayers for the sick.

Despite this being my first time to make such a hospital visit, the little prayer service went smoothly, and afterward we chatted for a while. Before I left, my friend thanked me for coming, especially for the prayers and communion. I can still hear her voice these many years later. "You're very good at this, you know, Maryann."

"At what? It's just a visit."

"No. It was more than that. It was a blessing, and you should do this for others."

I thought that was very nice of her to say, and I was truly glad that she'd found the visit so beneficial, but I didn't think much more about the last part of what she said, until a few weeks later. There was an announcement at church that a hospital ministry program was starting. Anyone who was interested could come and find out more about it during an evening meeting scheduled for the following week.

Could I?

Should I?

Yes, Lord, I will tend your sheep.

So, I went to that first meeting and many more afterward. Initially, we were trained by a woman who had been a hospice chaplain. She gave us books to read on this special ministry and told us the things we should, or shouldn't, do. Primarily that our role was to show the love of God to the patients we visited through prayer and holy communion. We were cautioned about getting too involved with families—something I always struggled with—because that kind of close involvement could be so traumatic when patients died. Another potential problem could arise if there were no clear boundaries as to what we would do, and some families might take advantage.

In addition to the training, we had weekly meetings to share our experiences and debrief, which was always so helpful. Because we were entering into such emotionally-charged situations when people were sick and/or dying, it was important that, after the hospital visits, we not keep our own strong feelings to ourselves. Sharing those experiences with other members of the ministry group was a good way to process how they were affecting us, and, in listening to how others handled situations, we learned ways to improve our own ministry.

I was part of that hospital ministry group for about seven years, and every moment was a blessing.

What you will read in the pages of this book are stories from the many years I tended the sheep through hospital ministry as a volunteer. Then later as a hospital chaplain, working full-time in a hospital in Omaha, Nebraska and part-time in another. Some of these stories were first written for a column I wrote for the Texas Catholic Newspaper when I lived in the Dallas area and did the volunteer work. Others came from experiences I had in Omaha. Those were first shared in a blog that had the same title as this book. I'd decided to write the blog as part of a lead-up to the first hardback release of my suspense novel, *One Small Victory*. Because grief issues are an integral part of that story, my publisher thought it would be a good way to create some early interest in the book.

Many of the following stories are taken directly from the columns and the blog with only a bit of editing for clarification purposes and to make smoother transitions from one to the other. While many of the stories deal with grief issues, some do not, but they are all connected by the thread of ministry. All of the names from the hospital stories have been changed to respect the privacy of the patients and staff and to make sure the HIPAA police don't come after me.

The last section of this book focuses on my own experiences with grief and how I struggled with them, despite all my training and the insights I'd gained helping others. So much of this grief stuff is so dramatically different when looking at it from the outside. A concept I didn't fully grasp until I was on the inside looking out.

Much of what you'll read in that last section is taken from blog posts that I wrote around the time of the deaths of my parents and my husband. I've always processed things through writing, so it is no surprise that I "wrote through" the most significant losses in my life.

This is in no way a definitive book on loss and the grieving process, and I'm certainly not trying to tell you how to walk your grief journey. It's just a book of stories, mine and others, that might provide some insights for yourself, whether you are in the midst of the pain of grief at the moment or not.

FIRST, A FEW FACTS ABOUT GRIEF

Hannah Siller, who is a counselor and life coach at Serene Life Consulting said recently on social media that grief doesn't happen in stages, "it's more like a grief yarn-ball, all sort of messed up and mixed up."

When I read that, I said, "Yeah. That's it exactly. Tangled."

Siller acknowledged that she didn't develop that theory on her own; she'd learned it in the classes she'd taken to get certified in trauma informed care. She currently has a Master of Science degree in counseling with an emphasis on trauma and crisis and is a doctoral candidate in psychology.

The common theories about a grief journey for a long time were that it happens in stages. The most referenced theory is from the Kubler-Ross model that lists the stages as: Denial, Anger, Bargaining, Depression, and Acceptance.

Denial is the most common first stage and often helps a person survive the initial loss almost in a state of shock, often described as feeling like one is walking through a fog.

Anger – Well, we all know what that is, and I'll share more about that later in this book.

Bargaining – Guilt is often a part of this stage, and I'd consider listing guilt as an actual stage. Depending on our circumstances, guilt can hang around for a long time like that proverbial unwelcome guest that shows up one day and won't go away. We start thinking of all the things we might have been able to do to prevent the death of that person we loved. Or we start thinking of all the ways we were unkind to that person, wishing we could time-travel and go back to do a retake.

Depression – This is when sadness may overwhelm us, and we want to withdraw from family and friends. Left unchecked, depression can lead to thoughts of suicide, making us wonder if life is really worth living anymore.

Acceptance – Coming to terms with the new reality, and life is okay again. Not in the sense that it is okay that we lost a loved one, but that we know we will be able to pull ourselves out of the deep black hole and go forward. There will be good days There will be bad days. And then there will be good days again. In this stage, it doesn't mean we'll never have another bad day—where sadness slams into us like a freight train. It's just that the good days will eventually begin to outnumber the bad days.

While most of us experience these stages after a significant loss in our life, there is no definitive order of when they will come, except perhaps for the first one. I think that one is pretty much set in stone. At least it is for me. My first reaction to the death of every person who was important to me has always been an immediate, "Oh, no," followed by days, or weeks, of feeling like I was living in an alternate universe. Things were happening around me, funerals, gatherings, and visitations, and I was part of it, yet not part of it.

Now, seven years after the most significant loss in my life, that of my husband, I've come to the conclusion that being in that alternate universe was where I needed to be those first few months after his death. Had I been fully living in reality, I would've experienced the pain of that loss so intensely, I might not have been able to bear it. As it was, when I did step into that reality, the pain was like a stab in the gut, but it didn't bring me to my knees. It hurt. It made me walk around crying a lot when I thought all the tears had been spent in previous weeks. It made me listless and restless, but it was bearable.

I don't think that reaction is unique to me.

~*~

It's important, too, to know that in addition to not going through the stages in any kind of order, we may not experience all of them. Some people only experience two or three. The theory that we go through all five stages in a chronological order, moving from the first to the fifth, has been disproven in more recent years by mental health professionals, and even Kubler-Ross has modified her model.

The truth is, nobody's grief is exactly like anyone else's, and there's no right or wrong to it at all.

Another important truth about the process is how important it is to have the freedom to tell our stories as often, and for as long, as we need to. I first learned that truth during my chaplaincy training. Too often, people are reluctant to speak openly about their grief beyond the first few days or weeks. A time period that seems to be socially appropriate.

They rationalize that decision by saying things like, "Others don't want to keep hearing the same thing over and over."

"We don't want to make them sad."

"Friends want to see us happy. See that we're over it."

"It's better to just keep quiet. Don't burden family or friends."

There are many other things that hold us back. Make us put on a brave face and say we're okay, but as one wise chaplain said to me when my husband had his first heart attack, "Maryann, when are you going to stop swallowing your feelings?"

That's why sharing is important. If you are grieving and sense that family and friends no longer want to hear about your sadness, I urge you to find a grief support group, or one close friend who doesn't tire of your story. It is so important for our physical and mental health to let those feelings out, so they don't fester inside and cause all kinds of physical problems.

~*~

When faced with the pain of someone else's, grief our instincts are always to try to make them feel better. That's such a common reaction. We don't want our friends to be hurting. We want to take the pain away. We want to give them some brightness and hope, anything to lift that dark cloud. So, we may try to offer them advice and encouragement, "It will get better." "He's in a better place."

Those well-meaning platitudes, as well as encouraging a

person to step away from their grief and their pain by focusing on what they still have, can all be more hurtful than helpful.

According to psychotherapist Megan Divine, who has written the book *It's Okay That You're Not Okay: Meeting Grief and Loss in a Culture That Doesn't Understand*, trying to make our friends and our family members feel better is actually counterproductive. She encourages people to enter into the pain with their friend and just acknowledge that their life pretty much sucks right now.

That was a difficult lesson for me to learn in my ministry because, as I mentioned earlier, I'm such a helper. When in a situation with a grieving person, it didn't seem like simply acknowledging the pain and letting the person be there in their sadness was helping. But finally, the realization dawned that a hurting person just needs acknowledgment.

"I see you."

"I hear you."

"I'm sorry that you're hurting."

And, when appropriate, an offer to hold them is often most welcomed. When I was going through the most difficult years of my grieving process, hugs, especially those that were heart to heart, seemed to bring me the greatest comfort. No words were spoken. No platitudes were tossed at me. Just a warm embrace.

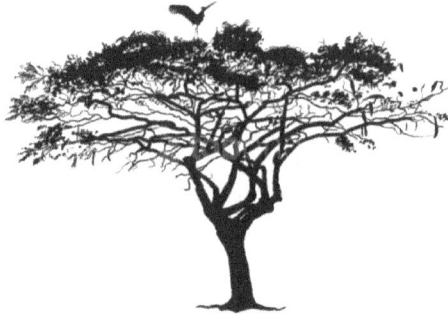

TESTED BY FIRE

My first experience with the death of a patient came when I was a brand-new member of the hospital ministry group at our church. A young man with leukemia belonged to our parish, and I was assigned to visit him in the hospital. That wouldn't be too bad. I could stop by on Sunday and bring him communion and maybe visit a little if he was up to it. No fuss. No sweat. Easy on the emotions.

At the time, the young man was receiving treatment that appeared to be working, so the plan was that he would go home and rejoin his young wife and children in a couple of weeks. Then I'd have a positive story to share with the rest of the group when we met for support and debriefing. Maybe we could even invite Hallmark in to make a commercial.

Why is it that when we think we have it all figured out, God, in His or Her infinite wisdom, throws the proverbial monkey wrench and all at us?

One day, several weeks after my last visit with this young

man in the hospital, the head of our ministry program called to ask if I would visit him at home. The treatments had stopped working. He was dying. He had asked for someone to come and bring him communion, and since I already had a connection to him, it would be good for me to make the visit.

Gulp! What happened to the Hallmark moment?

I went. But I'm not sure I was a whole lot of help to the family. I wasn't prepared for this sudden turn of events, and I wasn't sure how I could represent a God at whom I was a bit pissed. It was totally unfair that this man was dying, and I wanted to rail against a God who would let that happen. (Okay, I was a lot pissed.)

Looking back now, I have to smile. I'd forgotten how green I was at tending His sheep, all this and how unwilling I was to enter into that tough arena of death. It was obvious that in those early years of hospital ministry, I had a whole lot to learn about why bad things happen to good people and God's part in all that.

The experience with that young man was almost the end of my association with hospital ministry. After he died, I swore I wasn't going to do it any more. It was too hard. I didn't want to get attached to another patient and possibly have to watch them die.

That was my plan, but again, God had another one in mind. He/She introduced me to Rene.

KNOCKED OFF MY HORSE

I was a few weeks into my "I'm never going to do this again" attitude about hospital ministry, when I received a phone call from the chaplain at the local hospital. There was a woman in the ER who had just been told her nineteen-year-old daughter had a brain tumor and was going to die. Could I come? The lady was Catholic and needed someone from her faith to be there with her. I'd almost forgotten that I'd volunteered to go for Catholic patients in emergency situations some time earlier when the Chaplain had asked our group if there was anyone willing to do that.

I hadn't been called in a long time.

But now.

Even in the middle of the night.

How could I say no?

At the hospital, the Chaplain took me to an exam room in the ER where I saw a woman, Wilma, in the middle of the space amidst the clutter of abandoned medical equipment and scraps of plastic, and gauze and tape littering the floor. She was just standing there. Alone. Hands twisting in fear and anguish. Tears streaming down weathered cheeks. The bed was gone. Oh, my God, I thought. I'm too late. The girl is dead.

The chaplain introduced us, then left us alone. Wilma told me that they had taken her daughter, Rene, to surgery. The doctors were going to try to reduce the swelling in her brain caused by the tumor, but there was only a slim chance she'd make it through the ordeal of the surgery.

Faced with Wilma's naked fear and anguish, I wanted to run out the door, but I steeled myself and stayed. One of the biggest concerns Wilma had was that Rene might die without baptism. She explained that Rene's father was not Catholic and had refused to have the kids baptized, even though she'd begged him.

Was it possible to have her baptized now? Not just the emergency baptism, but a real one with a priest?

That was a big ask, and probably crossed some of those boundaries that we'd been told to keep during our volunteer training, but I couldn't ignore the desperation in her voice and her eyes. So, I said I'd see what I could do.

First, I called my husband to see if he would come to do the baptism. "If she specifically asked for a priest," he said, "she might not be comfortable with baptism being performed by a deacon."

The order of Permanent Deacons was still fairly new in the Catholic Church, and not everyone embraced them as members of the clergy or fully understood their role, despite the fact that the men are ordained. They can function in many roles that the priest does, preaching and administering sacraments, with the exception of Reconciliation (confession) and consecrating the Eucharist.

Because of the fact that so many people still didn't understand what functions a Deacon was authorized to perform, my husband said it would be better to see if our pastor would be willing to do the baptism. Fortunately, we were blessed to be in a parish with a pastor who took the call from Jesus to "tend My sheep" very seriously, and he agreed to come to the hospital.

It also helped that by then, it was no longer the middle of the night. Willingness is sometimes easier in daylight.

As soon as Rene came out of surgery, we went into the recovery room and the priest performed the baptism. Since I was the only other Catholic in the room, besides her mother and the pastor, I was named as her godmother.

Several days later, much to the doctor's surprise, Rene woke up and appeared to be just fine. Wilma called to tell me the good news, so I went by to visit a couple of hours later. After I walked into the room, Wilma started to introduce us, and Rene said, "I know who you are. You're my godmother."

I was incredulous. "You know?"

"Yes. I met you when I was baptized."

Considering the fact that she'd been in a medically induced coma when the sacrament had been administered, that revelation was incredibly hard to grasp. I don't think I could respond for a full minute, and even Wilma was speechless.

That was my St. Paul moment. You know, knock me off my horse to get my attention. I guess like St. Paul, I needed more than just a gentle nudge.

I THOUGHT I KNEW IT ALL

After my last visit with Rene in the hospital, I was sure that would be the end of our association, but something about her tugged at my heart, so when her mother asked if I would visit at home, there was no hesitation.

After fully recovering from the surgery, Rene decided she wanted to become a full member of the church, so, with the support of our pastor, I started going to her house once a week for informal catechism classes in preparation for her to make a full profession of faith. Not knowing how long she might live based on the doctor's prognosis, our pastor had recommended that I do a condensed version of a year-long journey that people take to become Catholic.

During those classes, we spent some time studying the Bible, as well as church history. Then during one session I wanted to introduce her to a bit of theology. I told her that the simplest definition of the word is "knowledge of God," and that one of the purposes of the practice of a religion is to deepen our knowledge and understanding of God. To be aware of His presence in our lives.

So, what would she like to learn about Jesus?

"Oh, I already know about Him," she said. "He was there in the hospital with me. We talked and He said I was going to be all right."

Here was another revelation that left me speechless for a few moments, and I couldn't help but think, "Wow! What other lessons will this young lady teach me?"

BLESSING ARE SOMETIMES SAD

While Rene was amazing me with her simple theology and delighting her family with her recovery, the doctors continued to be cautious about celebrating. Even after weeks of radiation, followed by a CAT scan that showed the tumor was gone, the neurologist told the family that this could only be a temporary victory. The kind of tumor Rene had rarely disappeared forever. There could still be cells lurking in her brain, ready to grow again.

Rene dismissed the doctor's negative prognosis and resumed her normal life, taking a few college classes, visiting with friends, and going to church. She'd named the tumor "Herman" and said she was convinced the radiation worked because she'd told Herman to "get the hell out of my head.

"And he did," she finished with the most confident smile.

Over the next few years, I didn't visit as often as I had been. I was busy with my family and my work, so what time was left for volunteering went to other people who needed support. Rene was busy, too, with her classes, as well as spending time with friends and family. When we did have a visit, I was always incredibly impressed with her child-like delight in life. Even today, I smile when I think of the way her eyes would sparkle with that delight, and how she'd laugh as she shared a joke or a funny story.

Herman stayed away for five years—four and a half years longer than the doctor had predicted—and when he came back, it was with a vengeance. By the time Rene was showing any symptoms, the tumor was larger than it had been originally and surgery was not even an option. They could try radiation again, but that might only buy her an extra few months.

She was pissed about that. She was also one of the few people I've met who openly expressed feelings of anger. She said a few nasty things to God about allowing this to happen to her, and her mother was horrified. "You can't talk to God like that."

"Actually, she can," I said. Then I told Wilma what a very wise woman had said to my daughter when a close friend's child had been killed. My daughter was angry that God had allowed that to happen, and this woman told her to go into her room, close the door, and tell God in no uncertain terms how she felt.

"But I'm mad," my daughter said. "I want to say ugly things."

"That's okay," the woman said. "God can take it. He's got strong shoulders. And He'd rather you yell at Him than turn away."

Over the next few weeks, I helped Rene and her mother prepare a memorial service. Rene picked out a couple of readings from the Bible, as well as asking for a particular song and a spiritual reading. The family, who had by then come to understand the role of a Deacon, wanted my husband to conduct the service, and his homily was focused on what a blessing Rene had been in our lives, as well as all of the things we'd learned from knowing her and sharing the past few years with her.

I was incredibly sad that Rene would not have the future she'd so desperately hoped for. She didn't finish college. Even though she'd made a provisional profession of faith, she didn't finish the instructions to make a formal one so she could receive the Sacrament of Confirmation. But she did accomplish so much in those four and a half years by showing us all how to accept what life throws at us.

Most importantly, she showed us how to live with great joy and how to die with grace and dignity.

NOTE: The names used in the stories about Rene are the real ones. After she died, I asked her mother if I could write these as columns for The Texas Catholic newspaper. Wilma gave me permission and said the names could be used. She wanted people to know about her Rene.

WHY BAD THINGS HAPPEN

One of the questions I am inevitably asked when talking to people about situations like Rene's is, "Why?"

"Why would a loving God take a young woman like that?"

Well, actually, God didn't do it. The tumor grew in her head without any help from Him at all. Good medicine and positive thinking kept it at bay for a long time, but it was inevitable that it would come back.

"But wait, what about miracles? Couldn't God have done a miracle here?"

Well, actually, yes. I do believe in miracles. And maybe it was a miracle that Rene had almost five good years instead of only six months. But that is only speculation. I think we can put an interpretation to almost anything after the fact.

And the fact is, God doesn't make things happen to people for whatever reason. He created us and the world we live in—at least some of us think so—but He turned control over that world to us. He could intervene on our behalf, and at times has done so, but most of the time He lets us chart our own course. He is not sitting up in Heaven with a computer keeping track of how good we are—I think it's only Santa and the Easter Bunny who do that—so He can bring down a terrible sickness on those who are sinning.

Too many of us grew up in religious experiences where we learned that we had to be good to please God, and in some way that started to equate to "Be good so nothing terrible happens."

However, as Rabbi Kushner points out in his book, *Why Bad Things Happen to Good People*, personal tragedy is not linked to personal morality or our behaviors. After the death of his son, Kushner came to this realization: "I had to leave behind the idea that if you're good, God rewards you. It took me years to come to the understanding that God does not send the problem, God sends us the grace to handle the problem."

It is from Kushner that I learned about the workings of natural law that operates with no moral judgment. He believes that natural law is blind to good or bad human behaviors, and God does not interfere with that natural law. God does not intervene to save good people from earthquake or disease and does not send these misfortunes to punish the wicked.

Does that mean that we should stop being good? Or stop praying for miracles? Absolutely not. We should always be good to mirror God's goodness and love, and I believe that God is dispensing miracles all the time. It's just that sometimes the miracle isn't what we asked for.

Sometimes the healing that we pray for isn't a physical healing, but a spiritual and emotional healing. And the worst thing that can happen is to be told that the physical healing didn't happen because our faith was not strong enough.

That happened to a friend of mine. One of her sons had spina bifida, a most severe neural defect, and when the

Charismatic movement started in the Catholic church, a group in our parish said they would pray for healing for him.

"A complete physical healing?" she asked. "Is that even possible just by praying?"

"Of course," they assured her.

My friend was, and still is, a woman of deep faith and spirituality, so she joined that group in praying for her son, but he did not miraculously throw his crutches away and walk one day. In fact, most days he had to use a wheelchair to move around.

In tears, my friend went back to the prayer group and asked, "Why?"

"Because your faith wasn't strong enough."

Words cannot express the depth of her devastation. The judgement of that group rocked her to her core, and it took years for her to stabilize again.

It also soured any interest I might have had in joining that prayer group.

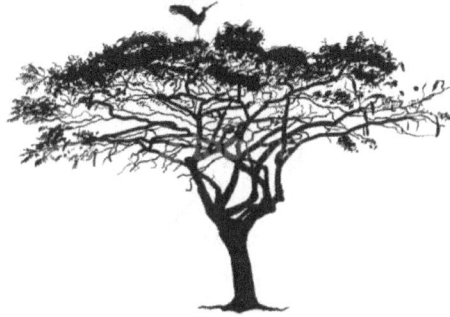

TURNING A HOSPITAL
MINISTER INTO A CHAPLAIN

When I moved to Omaha, Nebraska from the Dallas area, I wanted to continue my hospital ministry, so I called the closest hospital to see if I could volunteer there. They had a much larger Pastoral Care Department than the hospital in Texas, and the hospital also happened to be a training center for chaplains.

The very nice man, "Steve," who took my call, told me that in order to work, even as a volunteer, in any pastoral-care capacity at the hospital, I would have to complete at least one unit of Clinical Pastoral Education (CPE). My informal training through the hospital ministry organization at the church back in Texas didn't count. Nor did my years of experience. Both of those, and the fact that my husband was an ordained Permanent Deacon in the Catholic Church, would qualify me to enter the CPE program, but it wasn't enough to let me volunteer.

I'll admit it. I had a bit of an attitude about that and fumed most of the afternoon. Who was he to discount what I had done? I was trained by a woman who had years of experience with Hospice. And didn't he know I was a good person and only wanted to help people?

Actually, I think he did. And when I was able to let go of my attitude and sign up for that first unit of CPE, I started to understand. To be a chaplain, it takes more than being a good person, and we are not there to help people in the way most people think of helping. Chaplains see to the spiritual needs of the patients, whether that be in just sitting and listening, praying when appropriate, contacting their pastors, or just being a reflection of God's love in how we respond to those spiritual needs.

When I think about the first few months of that initial unit of training, I cringe remembering all the poor people I tried to "help." Steve was the CPE supervisor, so I met with him weekly to debrief and go over reports on my visits. I would feel so smug because of things I did to help patients, and Steve was quick to point out that wasn't my role. "You aren't here to 'fix' things," became his typical response to me, until I finally started to get it.

I went on to take three more units, which then qualified me to work first as an on-call chaplain, then part-time, and finally full-time for several years. Those were years filled with so many incredible experiences that I'm so very grateful for, and I'd almost let it all slip away because of my hurt feelings at not being immediately embraced into a new community of hospital ministers.

Once, after I'd been working full time for a couple of

years, I was sharing the end-of-day briefings with one of the other chaplains I'd grown particularly close to, and she remarked, "Every day is filled with so many blessings, they're almost enough to pay for the work. But don't tell our boss I said that. The paycheck comes in handy."

I had to agree on both counts. Our days were filled with wonderous encounters during which we could feel the grace of God working, but still, our meager bank accounts appreciated the financial infusion at the end of the week.

SHALL WE SING?

One of the areas I served during my CPE training was Rehab Day Services, housed in a large room furnished like a home with comfy chairs, a dining table, flowers, and artwork. Patients who had suffered head trauma from accidents or strokes, and had completed the in-hospital rehabilitation, would come for outpatient rehab and spend their down time in Day Services.

During lunch, there could be as many as ten patients gathered around the large table sharing a meal, and Jean, the director, would always encourage them to talk about their successes, as well as challenges and frustrations with their various therapy sessions.

Steve, my supervisor, thought it would be good for me to go to Day Services at noon to bring some spirituality to the gathering.

Ha.

There was so much spirituality already there, I wasn't sure what I was supposed to do.

They didn't need me to lead them in prayer before the meal. They already did that.

They didn't need someone to listen to their fears and frustration. They had open sharing after the meal, and it quickly became clear that they were already "chaplain" to each other; encouraging those who were struggling and celebrating with those who'd achieved a new milestone.

So, for the first few visits I sat and ate with them, joining in the conversations when appropriate, but always letting the patients have the floor, so to speak. Then one day, as lunch was winding down, someone started to sing while clearing the table. Several others joined in on a sweet version of "Amazing Grace" When I saw how the music brightened the faces of those who were a bit down that day and calmed the nervous jitter of others, I realized what I could do for them.

I could bring my guitar, and we could sing.

So, I did.

And we did.

To some amazing results.

When the music happened, I thought it was all about brightening their day, making them feel better, but we accomplished so much more.

THE MAGIC OF MUSIC

One of the patients at Day Services was a young man who had been in an automobile accident and had a severe closed-head injury. After the accident, he'd been in a coma for weeks, followed by weeks of inpatient rehab. Since I can't use his real name, I'll call him Dave.

Prior to his accident, Dave had been in a band with some other high school buddies, and he wrote much of the music. According to friends, the band was quite good and had actually played a few gigs, with hopes of more to come. Unfortunately, the accident had dashed those hopes, but Dave still liked to sing and would occasionally attempt to play my guitar.

One day, while I was strumming through the usual warm-up exercise I do right after tuning my guitar, Dave focused on the music. When I stopped, he asked me to keep playing the song. "It's not a song," I told him. "It's just a little riff I do."

"But it's a song," he said.

"Okay, sing it."

He did, adding a melody and lyrics to the chords as if he was reading it all from a piece of sheet music.

He sang that song every day for a week, with only slight variations in the melody notes, but wide disparity in the words due to his short-term memory difficulties. So, I got the idea to tape him singing and send the tape to my son in Texas who writes music. (This was before the magic of smart phone recording and instant sharing.) "Do you think you could write out the music?" I asked my son. "Smooth out the rough edges of the melody and fill in missing lyrics?"

My son didn't hesitate. "Sure."

A few weeks later, I was able to gift Dave with a tape of his song, as well as sheet music. He was thrilled. He still couldn't remember thelyrics from day to day, but he loved the idea of having his song.

One day his father told me, "That was the best thing anyone has done for my son in a long time. He listens to that tape every day on the way home from the hospital."

Other clients in Day Services had certain songs they wanted me to play week after week, and I thought that all the music was doing was making them happy for a little while. I had no idea that it was actually helping them physically.

I knew of the benefits of music therapy programs but had always thought of them as good for the soul, more than the body. But the director of the Day Services said that the music was helping, especially in Dave's case. "The music is physiologically beneficial to people with brain injuries," she said. "It helps the patient's brain to make new synaptic connections that compensate for those broken in the accident that caused the brain injury."

Even today, over twenty years later, it still thrills me to know that my meager musical talent was able to have such a positive impact.

If you'd like to know more about how music is helping patients with all kinds of brain injuries, there are great resources on the Internet, including an article on the Dana Foundation Website:

https://dana.org/article/how-music-helps-to-heal-the-in-jured-brain

ANOTHER GIFT OF MUSIC

During the time that we lived in Nebraska, my husband and I made frequent trips to Arlington, South Dakota. That's where my longtime girlfriend, Jan, lived with her parents, who, during my troubled youth, took me in and helped me become a better person than I was on track to be.

While I was living with them, it was too cumbersome to address her parents using their family name, or to always use the formal title of Mr. and Mrs. At that time, it was also disrespectful to call our elders by first names, so we came up with the idea that I should just call them Mam and Sir. That seem to satisfy us all, and after many years those titles became incredibly dear to me, as did the couple.

Fast forward quite a few years to after Sir had died from cancer, and my girlfriend Jan had given up on the promise she'd made to keep her mother, who had Alzheimer's, home with her. Mam's Alzheimer's had progressed to the point where she was totally unmanageable, hardly sleeping and prone to wandering at night, and Jan was getting no rest, which was seriously affecting her health. She finally had to make the difficult decision to put her mother in a nearby care facility.

When my husband and I could make a trip north from Omaha, Jan and I would make a special point to visit Mam. Remembering how her mother loved for me to play the hymns that she treasured, Jan asked me if I would bring my guitar. "You know how Mom always liked to hear you play and sing."

I was more than willing to share the music with Mam, and when we visited, the activities director at the facility would also bring some of the other clients in. They were folks who were mobile and compliant, so she'd bring them to the common room where they could also listen to the music. What a joy it was to see the faces light up with pleasure and recognition.

Where words and pictures and visitors failed to stimulate a bit of recognition in those people whose memories were failing them, the old hymns made connections. Often the clients would start to sing along, as a long-ago memory rose to the surface.

One of Mam's favorite hymns—the one that she never failed to ask for on visits made years ago when minds were still clear—was "In the Garden." So, it was that hymn that I played and sang whenever Jan and I went to see Mam.

On most of those visits, Mam would sit quietly while I sang, never joining in. Then one day I saw a smile of recognition slowly lift her lips, then she started to sing a few words, almost in a whisper. When the song ended, a tear ran in a slow trail down her wrinkled cheek, and that image will forever be embedded in my mind. In her expression and that tear, I saw enjoyment, remembrance, and maybe even an acknowledgment of her loss.

None of the articles or books I've read about the benefits of music therapy have included anything as profound as, or had the impact of, that moment.

MARYANN MILLER

GONE FISHIN'

Sometimes ministry takes strange turns. One wouldn't necessarily consider fishing a ministry, but in the case of Mr. Charles, it was.

Mr. Charles, a retired Presbyterian minister, was one of our neighbors in Omaha, and about a year after his wife died, he was diagnosed with leukemia. It was not the virulent leukemia that kills so many young people, He had Chronic Myelogenous Leukemia, which is a slow-progressing form of the blood cancer and is very treatable for several years.

I first met Mr. Charles when I was out walking my dog, and we passed by his corner lot, where he had a bountiful garden in the spring and summer, sharing his vegetables with anyone who would like some. He was one of the few neighbors who would be outside no matter what the weather was like, and we would often chat for a few minutes. He was intelligent and widely read, and had a formal way of speaking. He was thrilled to find out that my husband was a minister and that I was a chaplain, finding a common bond in shared ministry.

When I'd stop to visit, some of our other conversations revolved around fishing and the great walleyes that could be found in lakes north of us, although Mr. Charles preferred the trout at a lake much closer. One day, he told me how much he missed fishing, and I was surprised to find out he was no longer going out.

"Why not?" I asked.

"I used to go with my friend, but he died some time

back."

"Oh, I'm sorry," I murmured.

"My children, you see, they don't want me to go fishing by myself, especially now that I'm sick."

He had a son in California and a daughter in Texas. They visited two or three times a year, but weren't available for regular fishing trips.

Over the next week or so, Mr. Charles talked about fishing a couple more times when I stopped on my daily walk, and it finally hit me. Maybe he was really grieving for this loss in his life as much as the loss of his wife and his ministry. And maybe he was sending a silent wish, so one day I said, "Mr. Charles, would you like to go fishing with me sometime?"

"Oh, I thought you would never ask."

"But why didn't you just ask me?"

"Because a black man cannot invite a white woman to go fishing," he said. "That is the way I was raised. I could never be that forward. But there is nothing in that code of conduct that says I cannot accept your invitation."

So, for the next year, Mr. Charles and I went fishing about once a week in prime fishing times, stopping only when winter snowed us in.

Sometimes, we'd talk about the beauty and bounty of God, and other times we'd discuss social issues, or books, or whatever topic struck our fancy. Those conversations would always be on the drive to and from the lake, however. The time at the lake was spent in quiet contemplation of the warmth of the sun, the gentle splash of water against the dock, the screech of a gull, or the drone of a curious bee circling our can of soda.

Did we catch fish? Sometimes, but actually, catching a fish was never a criterion for measuring the success of a fishing trip. He'd made that clear on the first trip, asking if I had to get a fish on the line to be satisfied with a fishing trip.

"It doesn't matter," I replied. "I'm always just happy to be outdoors."

He nodded and smiled. Obviously, that was the answer he was hoping for.

The next summer, deteriorating health kept Mr. Charles at home, and his children came to visit more often. One day when I saw his daughter out tending to the garden, we stopped to chat. She told me then how much those outing to the lake had meant to him the previous year. "He talked about it a lot when we were on the phone last summer," she said. "So, thank you for making my father so happy."

I nodded. Words could not get past the lump in my throat.

WE SHOULD NOT DIE ALONE

One of my specialties as a hospital chaplain was dealing with crisis situations in the ER or ICU. During the years of hospital ministry in Texas, I'd been at a number of emergencies, and those experiences taught me a lot about myself. Primarily, that I've always been cool under pressure, which was an asset when dealing with grieving families that have emotions exploding all over the hospital room, or families facing tough choices, again with emotions that are out of control.

Sometimes I'd have to try to contain the wild, demonstrative grief that had people flailing over gurneys and falling to the floor. Other times, my service would entail standing quietly and holding a hand while someone died with no family present.

That happened often when family members had been keeping vigil for days and days, and just stepped out for a short break. Almost as if the dying person wanted to make that transition from life to death without family members in the room.

But on rare occasions it was because family members didn't care to be present for whatever reason.

One of the ICU nurses had a particularly hard time dealing with that kind of situation and called me one day in tears. A patient, who had an untreatable lung disease and had been on a ventilator for several weeks with no hope of ever breathing without it, wanted the vent removed. She had two sons, who had seldom visited in those weeks, and they had different reactions when the nurse called to relay their mother's wishes.

The first son said that was fine, "But no, I don't want to come to the hospital when it happens."

The second son said, "I'm not fine with the vent being removed, and I'll come to the hospital with a lawyer, if need be, to prevent it."

These calls were made the day the woman made her difficult decision, and she'd indicated by writing on a tablet that she didn't want to delay. She'd been thinking about her situation, and the outcome, for a week and was ready.

"Do you want to honor what your younger son said?" the nurse asked the woman, while we all still stood in her room.

An emphatic shake of her head was the immediate response.

Even though the woman had already signed a do-not-resuscitate (DNR) order, the nurse thought we should have another document clearly outlining the fact that the woman countered her son's demand. Just in case he came with a lawsuit after the fact. The legal department from the hospital drew up paperwork, outlining her most recent request, and that document was brought to her room. It was read to her, and then she signed it, with the nurse and myself as witnesses.

Then there was another conference call to the second son, during which the doctor again explained that there was no hope of recovery for his mother, and we now had another legal paper explicitly stating that she wanted the vent removed.

Legally, there was nothing else the son could do, but, as the nurse said, if he cared that much about his mother to fight the removal of the vent, he could have cared enough to visit in the weeks she'd been in the hospital. She'd been so alone and so afraid during those weeks, only having hospital staff coming in her room. "Where was his caring then? Where is his caring now? Surely, he could come and be with her when she died."

Everything was done to make the woman comfortable and before the vent was removed, I had a short service for her with prayers I'd written based on her feelings and requests. The service was short. Purposely so. There was no need to drag the moment on for any of us.

Then the woman nodded. Per the protocols of vent removal, the nurse injected a large dose of morphine to make the woman comfortable, and the respiratory therapist turned off the machine.

It only took moments.

Then the woman was gone.

The nurse cried. The therapist cried. And I cried. Not because the woman died. Well, maybe a little. But more because of the weeks she'd suffered the physical and emotional pain of facing the end of her life without the support and comfort from her sons. We cried, too, for the fact that she had to die with strangers around her bed instead of those sons to whom she'd given life.

I'd never experienced such a disconnect in a family before, even the most dysfunctional families. There'd been lots of times I saw the "who loves Mom the most" dynamic play out as siblings vied to be the most important person there.

I'd seen children or husbands or grandchildren cry and beg a person not to die, creating quite a spectacle.

I'd been present at so many difficult moments for families, but I'd not seen that kind of disregard, and it hit me hard. My frustration and anger were so strong that I had to work a long time to let go of the feelings and my judgements of those sons.

It took a while for me to fully accept the fact that it simply wasn't my place to judge them. For weeks afterward when I thought of the woman and her sons, I'd get mad at them all over again. It was only through processing the feelings in group with my CPE supervisor and the other chaplains that I was finally able to let go.

NO TIME TO DIE

During my years of working in the hospital, I found it odd that some people seemed to be able choose the day they were going to die, and somehow it happened, while others kept choosing to go to no avail. It made me wonder why people desperate to leave the misery of their illnesses often hung on for months, sometimes even years, unlike a few who seemed able to bypass the waiting by sheer determination.

Such was the case of one woman who was diagnosed with liver cancer. Her cancer was stage three—certainly worth a bit of a fight for some people—but she opted not to have treatment.

Her family was distressed at this decision, and I was called in during one particularly emotional moment when her son was begging her to reconsider. I have to admit that I didn't agree with the woman's decision. She was only in her early seventies, healthy, and had a large, loving family. Given her circumstances, and the prognosis of treatment possibly giving her many more good years, I thought maybe she should consider giving it a shot. I certainly would.

Still, that wasn't my call. Nor was it her son's. It was hers. And I was getting better at stepping aside and letting it be about the patient.

So, my role as chaplain was to advocate for this woman and help the family accept the decision when they came to me for support.

Once her husband and children came to terms with her decision, she threw them another curve ball. She didn't want to go home to die. She didn't want to put them through the experience of having to care for her 24/7.

Again, I didn't agree with that decision. Some beautiful things happen in families when they share a death journey, and I thought she was being thoughtless in denying her children something they obviously wanted. Besides all that, her cancer was not that far advanced. The oncologist thought that even without treatment, she could live six months to a year before she started to decline.

Once again, this was not my call. It was her decision, and as long as her insurance would pay for long-term care in our nursing home, she could go there. Our medical social worker arranged for her transfer, but pointed out the fact that the woman only had coverage for sixty days.

Over the next two months, I visited the woman two or three times a week, and she continued to pray for a swift death. As the end of those sixty days drew near, she seemed unconcerned about the possibility of having to go home. During one visit, she told me that she was confident God would take her before insurance ran out. The fact that medically she was nowhere near that moment of transition from one life to another didn't deter her from that belief.

On the 60th day, I visited her to find her awake, alert, and not showing any medical indication that she would not be able to be released. Plans were already in place for her to go home the following day.

We talked about her impeding release, and I asked her

how she felt about that.

"It'll be okay," she said. "It won't be long before I go to my heavenly home."

I was sure she was referencing a time frame that contained weeks, if not months spent at home with her family, so imagine my shock when I found out the next day that she had died.

I wasn't the only one to be surprised.

During our daily discharge rounds in the oncology department the next morning, we were all astonished to read the report that the woman had died shortly before midnight the night before.

Those of us around the conference table; nurses, social workers, dieticians, and myself, were beyond shock. No way should that woman have declined so dramatically in twelve hours and then died.

After the buzz of our initial amazement died down, we realized it would be fruitless to try to figure out how that could have happened. As unbelievable as that situation was, we'd all simply experienced too many mysteries to try to figure out the why and how of one more medical mystery.

SPIRITUALITY ISN'T LIMITED TO CHURCH

One of the things I learned in my years of training as a chaplain was the difference between spirituality and religion. Most of us tend to believe that the two are the same thing, but they aren't. Spirituality and religion can be intertwined, and are for many people, but others have a strong spirituality without ever setting foot in a church.

For instance, there are the people who find great peace and contentment while sitting on the bank of a river or lake with a fishing pole in hand. My friend, Mr. Charles, knew that he was nurturing his spirituality at the lake in much the same way as if he were in church or at home reading his Bible. The same was true for my friend, Sir, another man who was close to the land and also loved to fish. Often, he would be at the lake while Mam was in church with their children, and the family was just fine with that. No judgements either way, which was a beautiful thing to see.

Farmers who work the land often say that they never feel closer to God than when they're out at the break of dawn to see a spectacular sunrise, or sitting on the porch to watch the sun go down in a glorious splash of color. I can attest to that. Not that I became such a great farmer when I lived out in the country, but every morning when I went outside, I'd be overcome with awe and wonder at the beauty created for our enjoyment.

We humans have something that separates us from the rest of the animals. Some people think of it as a soul, others refer to it as a "spirit center." Whatever we do in our lives that make us feel whole and worthwhile is somehow connected to that spirit center. And this need to feel whole and worthwhile is as vital to our well-being as food and water and the air we breathe.

In my years of working at the hospital, I met many people who found religious practice to be the best way to feed their spirits, but I also met a number of folks who were relieved to find out that God would not strike them down for not going to church. I did, however, encourage them to nurture their spirituality in some way, whether it be through music, art, nature, or relationships with people. And to recognize that through that, they were connecting with some power outside themselves, whether they called it God or not.

There were two situations that taught me a lot about this difference between religion and spirituality, and that the latter can be strong without the former, at least when it comes to organized religion.

Once I was called to our Surgery/Medicine floor to visit a man who'd been injured in a motorcycle accident. His injuries weren't life-threatening. In fact, he might go home in a day or so after being watched for concussion. The nurse said the man was a little belligerent and maybe I could smooth his feathers.

Ha. Death I could deal with. Belligerence was another matter, but I went anyway. That was my job.

The door to the man's room was wide open, so I knocked, told him who I was, and asked if I could come in.

"I didn't call for no chaplain." He crossed his arms over his chest in a gesture I was well acquainted with.

"I know. I just thought we could visit a minute if that's okay."

"I don't need no God stuff," he said.

I chuckled. "Okay. No God stuff."

He looked at me for the first time since I'd knocked. "Suit yourself."

The man had tattoos covering both arms. Really nice skin

art as it's called today. Back then it was still referred to as ink. I commented about how pretty the images were, and he gave me another look. There was one image in particular that caught my eye, a rose with some lettering. I asked him what that stood for, and he proceeded to tell me about this bike club where he was a member. They held camps for disadvantaged kids every summer, and did a lot of mentoring throughout the school year.

For the next fifteen or twenty minutes we talked about that outreach his club did, as well as what kind of bike he had. The fact that on several occasions I'd ridden my father's old Harley, seemed to surprise and impress him, and stimulated more conversation.

The more we talked, the more animated he became, and his posture relaxed. No more arms crossed over his chest to hold me out.

Before winding the visit down, I told him, "That's your spirituality."

"What? I don't go to church."

So, I told him the difference between religion and spirituality. "Church is important to me for fellowship and shared beliefs. But that isn't for everyone. You obviously have fellowship and shared beliefs with the other members of the club."

He was quiet after that, but I could sense that he was processing what I said.

At that point I could have just left, but something prompted me to do one more thing. I wasn't sure what his response would be, but asked if he'd like to pray together.

He didn't respond right away, but I just felt this grace

building in the room. To my surprise he said yes. "But you pray, I'm not good at it."

I didn't believe that for a minute, but I also didn't argue. I took his large, weathered hand in mine and thanked God for this time we had shared. For the blessing that this man was to me. And asked God to help this man see how special he was and how much God loved him for all the good he was doing for young people.

I swear there was a tear in the man's eye when I finished.

ANOTHER LESSON LEARNED

When visiting American Indians in the hospital, I learned about a different kind of spirituality. The hospital was located in an area of Nebraska that had a large population of Indigenous people, and it was always an enlightening and pleasurable experience to visit with patients from the native cultures.

I had several such encounters with a man who was in for a couple of weeks recovering from heart surgery and he taught me a lesson I've never forgotten. He talked about the ritual performed by every person who wants to enter the prayer tent. "There's a path leading to the tent," he said. "And at the beginning of the path is a large pole stuck deep in the ground. Before you can enter the tent, you have to stop at the pole. If you have a grievance with a brother, you must put that on the pole before you can come to pray with a clean heart."

That's a wonderful tradition and ritual, and I think of that every Good Friday service at our church when we are invited to come to kiss or touch the large wooden cross that's been carried in for the service, often by the deacon. To me, that's the Catholic way of leaving our grievances at the pole before going back to our pew to pray with a clean heart.

HEAR THE MUSIC

Even though I've never considered myself a poet, occasionally some lines of poetry will pop into my head, so I write them down. That happened now and then when I was working at the hospital, and one day I realized I was writing one for a patient, "Bob."

He was an elderly black man with a large, loving family and his illness dragged over a number of years, the last two keeping him almost completely bedridden. He had congestive heart failure, chronic obstructive pulmonary disease (COPD), and diabetes.

One of the great joys in Bob's life, besides his family, was music. He sang in his church choir, and one daughter said he sang around the house all the time. She could remember having family gatherings that turned into great music fests when she was young. Her father would lead them in singing all the popular songs, as well as church hymns.

During Bob's hospital stays we would sing whenever he felt up to it when I visited him, and often the sound of the music that drifted out of his room would draw other folks in for a chorus or two, including nurses.

To hear Bob sing "Precious Lord" was a tremendous blessing.

One time when I brought the young man, Dave, from Re-hab Day Services to sing with Bob, he cried. I can still see the smile that lit up Bob's face, despite the tears, and when the visit was winding down, he said, "That boy sings like an angel."

Bob's delight in music touched my heart in a special way, and I finally realized one day that the snatches of poetry in my journal had been inspired by him. And I knew this poem was for him.

HEAR THE MUSIC

Sing the song of life,
Take it,
Embrace it,
Carry it deep in your heart
Where the melody reaches out
And plays to the rhythm of your soul.

Dance the song of life.
Feel it,
Rejoice in it,
Let it carry your soul
To the far reaches of the heavens
Where God dwells.

When the song is ending,
Don't despair.
As the final note draws near,
Take it,

Embrace it,
Rejoice in it,
For the song never really dies.

THE GIFT THAT WAS BOB

When I was working in the hospital, there were many instances when I felt like I was benefiting more from visits than the patients were, and my visits with Bob definitely fell into that category.

In addition to the beautiful music that he so freely shared, I was also privy to his strong faith and unwavering trust. He never asked why God did this to him. The only "why" question Bob asked was why God didn't just take him. Why was he lingering for so long?

As I have said before, I don't think God is that actively involved in our dying. I know that many people believe that our day and time of death is preordained, but it is not a concept I've ever been able to embrace. Not that there's anything wrong with believing that God knows the time and day of our passing, it's just not part of my theology.

Therefore, my answer to Bob about why God had not taken him was, "I don't know."

After we sat quietly for a moment he said softly, "But I'm no good to anybody any more. I can't do anything."

That whispered pronouncement tore my heart and I struggled to maintain the boundaries and respond in a professional way, instead of pulling him into a hug and telling him how much I didn't want him to go.

I took a breath and said, "When I think of you and your goodness, I think of the blessing you have been to our hospital. You've been here so often in the past two years, almost everyone who works here has met you. Shared songs with you. We've met your wonderful faith-filled family. People who got that faith from you."

He clutched my hand and tears spilled down his cheeks. I squeezed back and finished, "You've been more than a patient here. You've been a gift to our hospital."

His life *graced* us.

Do Not Be Afraid

"Do not be afraid, I am with you.

I have called you each by name.

Do not be afraid, I am with you.

I have called you each by name.

Come and follow me

I will bring you home;

I love you and you are mine."

That's a verse from a hymn, "You Are Mine," which is one of my favorites. I always think of it when visiting with patients who are facing the end of life and suddenly the fear sets in. That was true with Bob. During one visit he admitted to me that even though he thought he was ready, he was afraid of dying. Like many people of faith, he occasionally had doubts about heaven and eternal life because those concepts defy rational thought, but he had trouble voicing those doubts. After all, people of faith are supposed to be sure.

"You're not alone in those concerns," I told Bob. "And it doesn't mean you've lost your faith. Remember how Jesus prayed in the garden before His death?"

Bob nodded.

"That prayer was wrenched from the same fear and doubt you're experiencing."

Bob thought about that for a long moment. Then he told me that one of his biggest fears was of the pain and discomfort he might experience in the dying process. He knew that as the COPD worsened it would become more difficult to breathe. "I'm so afraid of suffocating."

I let the admission just be there for a few moments, then said, "That is a scary prospect. But be assured that the staff here will do all they can to make sure you're comfortable."

That seemed to ease his concerns for the moment, and I sincerely hoped that Bob's ending wouldn't be filled with the agony he was so afraid of.

Several weeks later, Bob was back in the hospital, and now he could no longer sing because he couldn't draw enough breath to support music. Frequently, a very kind lady from housekeeping would come in and sing "Precious Lord" and Bob's eyes would light up. His lips would move as he silently mouthed the words, and I'd smile through the tears that misted my eyes.

Neither Bob or his family knew that this was to be his last visit to the hospital, but his condition continued to deteriorate.

His last few days were spent in ICU, where medications helped with the painful process of dying of asphyxiation, but it also numbed him to human interactions. That didn't keep friends and family away, however, and the afternoon he died, the ICU room was filled with the whole family, their pastor, and a few close friends. I offered to leave since he had so much support, but his daughter said, "No. You've been with him through it all. You should stay if you can."

I was on call that day, which meant I could have been paged to ER at any time, but the pager remained silent for the next hour.

Everybody took turns standing at the head of his bed to talk to Bob or to sing a song. I stood at the foot of the bed and waited, just marveling in the glory of this wonderful family and beautiful experience.

Then it happened.

There was a hush in the room. I looked over at Bob and saw his spirit lift from his body. It was so quick, I almost convinced myself I didn't see it, but the image of his smiling face is imprinted on my mind. The deep lines of fear and anxiety he'd worn for months had been smoothed by the most beatific smile.

A few days later, I shared that with his widow. "Really?" she asked. "You really saw his spirit."

"Yes. I wasn't sure at first. But oh, that beaming smile on his face. I'll never forget it. I think he knew he was going to Heaven. To be at peace."

Tears streamed down her face and she clutched my hand. "Thank you for telling me."

"I know that doesn't ease the pain of your loss, but I hope that knowing how he smiled on his way will bring you comfort. Maybe in time to come."

She nodded.

It was my great honor to be asked to deliver a eulogy at Bob's funeral. Unfortunately, the funeral coincided with my husband's first heart attack, so there was no question as to where I would be.

WILL THE REAL CHAPLAIN PLEASE STAND?

Perhaps because of my long association with hospital ministry, I've always been a fan of medical shows, and one of my favorites was ER. When the writers and producers added the character of a chaplain to the cast, I was delighted. Finally, more people would be able to see a chaplain in action, finding out that chaplains do so much more than stop by a room with a smile, a prayer, and a Bible. For people who watched the show, it would be a good introduction so they'd have familiarity before meeting a real chaplain for the first time in the midst of their own health crisis, or the crisis of a loved one— as long as the writers did their research. Since the writers seemed to go for accuracy on the medical side, I was hopeful the same would be true for this spiritual part of health care.

At first, I liked the new character and could relate to her somewhat offbeat and irreverent approach to the job, noting that she clearly made that all-important distinction between spirituality and religion to some of the patients. Not everyone gets that difference, so I applauded the series writers for doing their homework before creating this character.

That confidence faltered a bit when part of the storyline shifted to being more about her relationship with one particular doctor than about her job. I was disappointed at this shift in focus, but the rest of what was presented about her job still rang true for the most part, so I continued to cheer for her.

The cheering came to an abrupt halt during one episode when the chaplain fled from a patient who was asking her for forgiveness. The patient, who was a doctor, had worked in a prison as an executioner. In his later years, he came to regret what he had done and set out to seek forgiveness, believing that his deeds were so terrible there was no way God could forgive him unless he somehow made restitution first.

Driven by the need to assuage his guilt, this doctor spent a number of years seeking out the families of the people he executed to offer a gesture of restitution. Sometimes it was through a gift of money, and other times offering some other kind of assistance. Still, his guilt overwhelmed him, and now he was on his deathbed, terrified that he had no hope of salvation.

The chaplain was called in to help this man find peace, but she couldn't do it. Instead of entering the place where he was and giving him the assurance that God could forgive him and would accept his atonement, she countered the man's need for forgiveness. She kept trying to assure him that what he'd done was "just his job" and nobody needed to forgive him for doing something he'd been mandated to do by a state government and a judicial system. In desperation and frustration, he finally screamed at her to get out.

So, she fled.

Of course, this conflict added to the drama of the show, but in real life, the chaplain would need to put aside her personal theology and give the patient what he or she needs to be at peace. If that means going against a personal belief, so be it.

Early in my CPE training, I learned that what I would be doing in hospital rooms wasn't going to be about me and what I believe. It would be about the patient, and what he or she believes. I could share my theology, and did so at times, but more often I needed to work within the bounds of a patient's theology.

It is their heart and soul that needs to be touched during ministry, not mine.

ANGRY? NO, I'M NOT ANGRY

Anger is often one of the hardest emotions to deal with in the grieving process, especially when that anger is directed at the person who died. Every person who ever attended one of the grief support groups I facilitated found this the hardest emotion to talk openly about. They all said that even thinking it made them feel so guilty. "How can we be mad at someone for dying? It's not like they did it on purpose."

Still, it's normal to have this kind of anger, and if it is not expressed, it can create havoc on a person's emotional and physical wellbeing.

I remember one woman who talked every week about her difficulty with making coffee in the mornings. She and her husband used to have coffee together every morning, and, now that he was gone, she just couldn't bring herself to make the coffee. On the surface, this sounded like so many other stories of what grieving spouses could no longer do, but I sensed that there was something deeper that she was having difficulty facing. So, I gently prodded her to think about how she felt about the fact that he was no longer there to share that special time. I asked if she could possibly be angry, and she was quick to say, "No."

She also said that she was not angry at him for leaving her now solely responsible for the family, the house, the finances, and the cars. Although she did say that she was disappointed that he did not make more of an effort to put some things in better order before he died. But angry? "No. I loved him. How could I be angry?"

This went on for several weeks, and I think others in the group suspected there was another layer to all of this, but they were patient, as was I.

Then one day the woman came to group, and her whole demeanor was different. She stood straighter, had a smile, and was wearing makeup for the first time in months. After she sat down, she looked around the room and then announced that she'd finally made coffee that morning. When asked what the turning point was, she said that she had a "come to Jesus" talk with her deceased husband during the night. "I told him everything," she said. "Even how angry I am that he died and left me all alone."

We all laughed, then hugged her.

After that, we didn't see much of that woman. She came to group a few more times, but I think rounding that most difficult corner in her grief journey set her on a straighter path forward and she "outgrew" the need for a support group.

It's amazing how that can work.

As I write this, I can't help but think of a time when my husband helped a good friend let his anger rise to the surface. Our friends had just lost their five-year-old son to a horrible accident, and the father was so angry, he was pacing on the back driveway. The dark, angry feelings were so strong he couldn't be still, he couldn't stay inside, but he was unable to express them. My husband went out to be with our friend and goaded him until he finally let go. He destroyed their entire wooden fence while screaming his rage.

I don't advocate going to that kind of extreme, but I do advocate not burying that feeling, even though I find it so difficult myself to let that feeling out. I'm a great one to dig a deep hole and put things in it I don't want to deal with. Anger being a biggie. Probably because I grew up in a family that had no clue about healthy ways to express that particular emotion. Anger tended to erupt like some dormant volcano, and I would run to avoid the flow of lava. That impulse to run is even stronger when I'm running from my own red monster.

But like that friend told my daughter so many years ago, we can take that anger to God. He has broad shoulders. He can take it.

WILL WONDERS NEVER CEASE?

One day I was called to the ICU to help mediate a difficult situation. A woman, "Alice," wanted to be taken off the ventilator. She had suffered a heart attack the week before, but her prognosis was not dire. The cardiologist was certain she could be treated with medicine following the heart catheterization that had opened a blocked artery. It was during that procedure that Alice had been put on the vent—standard for any surgeries—but for some reason when the medical staff tried to remove the vent, Alice was not able to breathe on her own.

Alice was lucid and clear about her intentions. She didn't want to be kept alive on a vent, not even for another few days to see if the medicine to improve her pulmonary situation would start working. Her husband, a second husband and not the father of her children, was willing to abide by her wishes. One daughter was also willing to do whatever Alice wanted.

The rest of the family, however, was desperate to keep their mother alive, and that desperation was bolstered by the doctor's opinion that it was too soon to remove the vent and "give up."

This was a very dysfunctional family with a history of addictions and lots of unresolved issues. They all appealed to me to "talk some sense into my mother," and I had to gently tell them that wasn't my job. My job was to determine if Alice fully understood her decision and then be her advocate.

On the tablet provided for her, Alice wrote that she did understand that she would probably die when the vent was removed and she was ready. She asked me to pray with her and for her, and continue to pray for her children after she was gone.

We held a brief prayer service and the vent was removed. I stayed with the family for about an hour, but somehow Alice managed to hang on. I was called to another situation that took a couple of hours to resolve, and when I checked back, Alice was still breathing.

At the end of the day, I stopped by her room before leaving the hospital, and she was still breathing. Still not fully conscious, though, as she'd been given strong medication to ease any discomfort if she struggled to grasp air. She seemed peaceful enough, but I thought surely, she would be gone when I came back to work the next day.

Much to my surprise I found her still listed on the patient roster in the morning. When I went up to her room, I found her awake, alert, and very much out of danger. The doctor was amazed. The family was amazed, and even Alice was amazed.

MORE ABOUT ALICE

The dynamics of Alice's family were most unusual. There were four adult children, two men and two women, who all had problems of one sort or another, and Alice freely admitted that her lifestyle, and lack of skills as a mother, contributed in large part to the dysfunction. That, and an alcoholic ex-husband, who was the father of the four.

But in these later years, Alice had tried to make peace with her family, and with God, after finally finding a second husband who was life-giving instead of life-destroying. "Hal is so good to me, and to the kids, even though they aren't his."

She was particularly close to one daughter, "Katie," who had forgiven Alice for past mistakes and accepted the new husband. This particular daughter was more emotionally stable than the others, and had gone through some counseling to come to terms with her past and how it affected her. The other three seemed immersed in their dysfunction, and were not open to forgiving Alice or accepting her new husband.

That made visiting times at the hospital a bit of a challenge when more than one showed up at a time, and it wasn't a huge surprise to me that the people most willing to step aside for the demands of the others were Katie and Hal. They were also the only two in the family who had supported Alice in her wish to have the vent removed.

In an attempt to find some reason for "God not taking me," Alice wondered aloud if she needed to stay to bring some peace to her family.

"What do you think?" I asked her.

She shrugged. "I really don't know. But what other reason could there be?"

"There may not be a reason. Other than it just wasn't your time to go. But maybe this is a chance to bring some healing to your family."

She nodded, and when we prayed, her prayer was that God would open the hearts of her children so they could all accept Hal and make peace with each other.

During the prayer time, Hal would leave the room. He was a professed atheist, and I thought that was why he'd slip out to the hall. One day I asked him if he was offended by the prayer. "Not at all," he replied. "I know it's important to Alice, and I respect her faith. I just think it might be disrespectful for an atheist to remain in the room during a prayer."

Wow! I had no words, and even today I still find that most

interesting and profound.

Alice lived for three more years, but she was in and out of the hospital several times for complications of diabetes and respiratory problems. Each time she was admitted, I'd visit her and ask how the "family peace plan" was going. She would just shake her head, so we would pray some more.

Finally, the last time she was in the hospital, she told me that maybe the reason she was still hanging in had nothing to do with helping her children, as they all seemed to have the same problems they always had. I told her that these questions of "why" often have elusive answers, and if she'd had any joys in the past few years, perhaps that was reason enough to be alive.

A few months later, Alice died suddenly at home.

Then she got her answer.

ALICE'S LEGACY

When Hal called me to tell me Alice had died, he also asked if I would officiate at her funeral. I was honored to be asked, and because Alice and I had read a lot of Scripture together, I knew some of the readings that were meaningful to her. I also knew that she would want her funeral to be a celebration of her life, so that is what I focused on in planning the service.

I worked with Hal and Katie in the preparations to make sure that anything that they wanted would be included, and Katie arranged for someone to sing a couple of her mother's favorite hymns.

Because of Hal's professed atheism, I wasn't sure how all this religious stuff was going to go down with him, but he said it was okay. "This is for Alice. This is what she wanted."

So, the service started with "Amazing Grace" and a prayer, followed by two scripture readings. Then, I gave the eulogy and a reflection on the past three years of knowing Alice and how her life had blessed my life. I reminded her sons and daughters how much she loved them and how we had prayed frequently for their wellbeing. I asked them to honor her memory and her final wish by finding a way to be at peace with each other, and with Hal, because no matter what they thought of him, he did love their mother intensely.

Following my talk, I invited people to come up to share memories and reflections. After a few people spoke, Hal stepped up to the lectern. He briefly addressed some of the problems the family had been experiencing, and asked the children to take my words to heart.

Then he talked about how important prayer had been to Alice and how he had always respected that, even though he was not a man of prayer himself. Then he turned to where I was seated behind him and said, "What do you think, Chaplain? Should we say one more prayer for Alice?"

He took me by the hand and led me over to the casket. We stood there for a moment, and I couldn't speak over the lump in my throat. I could feel the silent expectancy in the room, but I still could not formulate words. Then Hal took a deep breath and said the most beautiful prayer.

Ah, Alice, that was your reason why.

TREASURES

One of the questions frequently asked in the grief support groups I facilitated was, "When is it time to clear out a loved one's belongings?"

What a loaded question, and it never failed to generate a myriad of responses.

Truth is, there is no "right" time. Or I should rephrase that and say there is a right time for every individual, and that person's right time may never be the right time for anyone else.

Many people theorize that it is not healthy to keep clothes and other items as they are just daily reminders of the loss. Because of that, they are quick to encourage "clearing things out and getting on with life."

But that is not necessarily what a grieving person needs.

A grieving person may need those things to touch and re-connect and remember for as long as it takes until they are ready to let go.

When a couple we know lost their five-year-old son in a tragic accident, some other friends cleared out the boy's room while the parents were at the funeral and took everything away, including furniture. The friends meant well, thinking they were doing the right thing by sparing the parents from the painful experience of sorting through his room, but they had no idea that facing the empty room was harder than facing all the boy's treasures.

The parents were too kind, and maybe still too numb, to

express anger at the friends' misguided help, but later the husband told me how devastated they were at the time. "There's not one thing left of our son," he said. "Just some pictures on the wall, and in some of our albums."

He took a deep shuddering breath then whispered, "I just wish I had something that belonged to him to hold on to."

Several months later, I was visiting and the father told me that he found a matchbox car in a far corner of his closet. "Paul must have left it there one day while he was playing. He liked to bring toys in the bedroom and watch me get ready for work. Somehow it ended up in the closet."

That little car became the father's most treasured possession.

ANGELS

At church one day, a man came up to our choir area after Mass and said to me, "You sing like an angel."

That was such a nice affirmation and I smiled and thanked him, while part of me wanted to say, "Wait, my singing isn't all that great. Pretty good maybe, but certainly not celestial. And I'm anything but an angel."

Still, his comment made me feel so good, and it reminded me of another man who called me an angel, specifically, his angel. I first met "Dick" when his wife was in the hospital. She'd just been diagnosed with cancer and was on our med/surg floor to have a port put in for her chemo treatments. Dick was terrified. In her room, he kept a running patter of positive comments and encouraging words, but later he came down to the Pastoral Services office and broke down. He cried, and between his tears he said, "She just can't die. She's young. I need her. I'm so afraid."

Earlier, while we were with her, he'd shown no sign of wanting to go to that dark place, and I was surprised when he shared it all in the private area of our offices. I was also honored that he trusted me enough to be that open. After all, we'd just met, and often it would take two to three visits, or more, to reach that level of trust.

There were no words needed from me at that moment, so I just rested my hand on his arm and let him cry. When the tears were over, he gave me a wan smile. "Sorry about weeping all over you."

"We have lots of tissues here in our office."

He smiled again, then said, "I'd better get back upstairs. Sherry will wonder where I am."

Dick and "Sherry" weren't strong religious people—I seemed to attract a lot of those kinds in my work, which was interesting. But they were deeply spiritual and very open to prayer. They just didn't always do that in a church.

Over a period of several months, Sherry was in and out of the hospital for treatments and setbacks, but then they finally got the word that she was in remission. I was delighted. As much as I enjoyed ministering to, and with, them, I always hated it when patients had to return.

Then one day I got a call in the office from a room upstairs. It was Dick. He'd heard me say the morning prayer that was a part of the normal routine in the Lutheran Hospital where I worked. We chaplains took turns greeting the day, the patients, and the staff with a short service every morning.

The first thing Dick said was, "I heard the prayer this morning and recognized the voice of our angel."

I responded that it was good to hear from him, and I was glad the prayer touched him. Then I asked if Sherry was back in the hospital. "No, he said. "I'm the patient this time, but it's nothing serious. In fact, I'll be going home tomorrow."

That was certainly good news after all the scary days and weeks and months the couple had gone through with Sherry's treatments.

Over the next year, the couple would come by the Pastoral Services office when they were in for routine checkups. It was always good to see them, especially since they both seemed to be doing so well physically, and there was a special closeness between them that was very evident. They were walking examples of the truism that while sometimes adversity pushes people apart, there are times it can strengthen a relationship.

When I resigned to move back to Texas, Dick and Sherry came to my going-away party and brought me a very special gift, a decorative piece with the words "You are an Angel" inscribed on it. I still have that cute artwork. It's hanging here on my office wall and reminds me daily of the blessing that couple was in my life.

While I don't consider myself an angel, I do believe in their existence, but I'm not so sure who had been the angel in all those years I worked as a chaplain.

ANOTHER PERSPECTIVE ON GRIEF

The following came in an e-mail from one of my cousins after she read some of my entries on the blog I did about loss. I liked what she had to say, so I thought it worth sharing:

I know I have never seen the spirit lift from a body, as you described in your blog, but I am certain it happens, and that there are those who are aware of it. Dying is a road we all must travel, and like you, I feel certain that most of us are apprehensive, to say the very least. I guess my father always tried to put things into perspective for me, as he would often say, "There are worse things than death."

I remember questioning that type of philosophy. What could possibly be worse than dying, of not existing anymore? When he explained his thinking, he told me that death is a release that we need when we are too sick to ever get well again. That relief and release will be welcomed at that point. I will never forget that conversation he and I had, even though it took me a few years, to see exactly what he meant.

Then there was the quote from *Thanatopsis, A View of Death* by William Cullen Bryan that we had to memorize in high school that tells us, "So live, that when thy summons comes to join that innumerable caravan which moves to that mysterious realm, where each shall take his chamber in the silent halls of death, thou go not like a quarry slave at night, scourged to his dungeon, but sustained and soothed by an unfaltering trust, approach thy grave like one who wraps the draperies of his couch about him and lies down to pleasant dreams."

One of my friends from high school is facing the prospect

of a "sudden death" from a heart problem that has taken away her ability to oxygenate her body. She is on oxygen 24/7 now after fighting it for several years. She is an RN, and a good one, so she knows too well what is happening. Because I think the world of this woman, who is a beautiful person inside and out, I wanted to do something to offer her some support, so one day I printed a copy of THANATOPSIS from my computer and mailed it to her. I also told her about some good books that covered death and near-death experiences of some ordinary people. She appreciated my trying to alleviate some of her anxieties.

That was the end of my cousin's message to me, but, reading about what she did for her friend, reinforced my belief that anyone, and perhaps all of us, can be ministers to each other, with or without formal training.

PLANNING FOR THE END

It is amazing the different ways that people respond to the dreaded words, "You have a terminal illness." Some panic and get hysterical. (I might just do that.) Others withdraw into a dark depression. Other's wage an intricate war, drawing up battle plans that rival any major military action.

Sometimes they continue that battle long past the time when winning is even a hope. Is that better than giving in to the inevitable? I don't know. I try always not to judge someone's coping mechanism, and sometimes pretending is the only way to keep from simply crumbling into a terrified heap.

On the other hand, there is something to be said for

accepting the inevitable. It affords time to take care of the business of one's life ending. I can't tell you how many widows in my support groups were struggling with the anger they felt at their husbands who didn't put things in order so the wife could carry on with financial and other matters. Surprisingly, that can still be a significant issue with couples where one or the other handles banking, investments, and household business. It would be so much easier for the person left behind if he or she were thoroughly briefed before their partner died.

Openly acknowledging the inevitability of death also affords time to take care of issues or problems in relationships. Nothing is harder on the patient, or the family, than to go through this kind of crisis with huge problems hanging over them.

While living is still happening, old hurts can be forgiven. Words that should have been spoken can still be said, and healing can take place.

For the families that don't have unresolved issues lurking in the shadows, the time left with a loved one can be used to start the grieving process and mark each moment in some special way. One family I knew had visitors write messages in a book that were then read over and over to the dying person. The book was then given to the next of kin after the funeral. Another family gathered frequently to sing and share memories of their loved one. For all of them, it was a time to treasure the person for one more day, one more minute.

It was always an honor for me to share these journeys with families, and I came to recognize that the gatherings, the memories, the singing, all made the going easier for the one who was dying.

Those experiences also helped me when my mother was dying, and I was able to be with her for her last few days.

PLANNING FOR THE SEND-OFF

There is something very special about funerals and memorials for people when they have worked with family to plan the services in advance. I've attended a number of those for friends who had picked all the scripture readings, music, and people to deliver the eulogy. Knowing that this had all been done in advance by the friend who had died, brought a special element to the ceremonies. It was like that person was actually with us that day.

The thought of pre-planning a funeral scares the bejeebers out of a lot of people. They think that if they actually put the plans on paper, they are somehow alerting the Grim Reaper and he will pounce. That is especially true with people who have been diagnosed with a terminal illness. But planning a funeral service will not hasten death. It merely gives a person some small measure of control in a situation where they have so little.

We have no say in what illnesses we might get. Well, okay, we can do some things to stay healthy. But even so, cancer, heart attacks, strokes, and other terminal illnesses strike almost randomly at times. So, the only control we have when we are looking at the stark reality of death is what happens afterward. We can decide if we want to be cremated or not. If so, where do we want our ashes to end up? Where do we want to be buried? What kind of service do we want?

Memorial services that celebrate a person's life have become very popular and appeal to a lot of people who are making these decisions. "I want people to remember me as having a good time and enjoying life," one patient said. "And I want a party afterward."

Some patients have told me that being able to make these decisions and plan for the "afterward" has made their last few weeks, or days, much more bearable. And family and friends attending services planned by the deceased have found comfort in the knowledge that their loved ones were part of the planning and that made the service more meaningful.

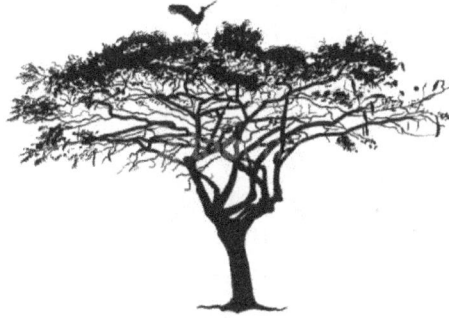

WE LOSE MANY THINGS

I used to think that grief only came after losing someone special—a grandmother, a mother, a father, a husband, a sibling, or a child. Their passing leaves a hole in our hearts and in our lives; a hole that we have to somehow learn how to live with. Most of us already know about the impact of losing people dear to us. We've walked that path of grief after someone has died, but we don't always realize that grief happens with other losses in our lives.

I certainly didn't understand that before I took my CPE classes. It was there that I was introduced to the importance of acknowledging the grief that comes from experiences like moving, for example. We go to a new home. A new place. And while that can be exciting on one hand, we're leaving something behind. The older home that holds so many memories of good times. Friends in the neighborhood that we may not see again. Perhaps a church home and community. Maybe a job we enjoyed and a "family" at work that was special.

THE MANY FACES OF GRIEF

When we move, for whatever reason, we need to let our feelings about leaving rise to the surface, so we can look at them and let them run their course. Just like we need to let the grieving happen when we lose a job or face a divorce. Divorce is the death of a relationship and extremely traumatic, especially when one partner doesn't want it.

There can also be grief associated with the death of a beloved pet. Some people scoff at the idea of grieving for a pet, but there are many more who understand completely. If we open our hearts and our homes to animals, their passing can have significant impact, leaving a different kind of hole in our lives.

I've been an animal lover my whole life, and there have been many dogs and cats who have graced my life for a time. When they passed on, the passing on was always so hard.

When I was a child, we were poor, so there was no money for veterinarians. We nursed sick or injured animals as best we could, and I was always devastated when our ministrations failed.

Once, in desperation, I carried a sick cat almost two miles to a veterinarian, asking if he could help. I had two dollars I'd been saving to buy some ceramic horses at the thrift shop on the corner of our street, but I told the doctor I'd pay him that two dollars.

I was about nine years old.

Unfortunately, the cat was too sick for any hope of recovery, so I carried her and my two dollars back home. She later died, and I buried her in the back yard.

Ironically, about nine years later, I got a job working for

that veterinarian, but he didn't remember the little girl with the two dollars.

It is now many years past the time I worked at that animal hospital, but I've never lost that deep affinity for animals. There has never been a time in my life that I have not had pets; sometimes just one cat or dog. sometimes more than one cat or dog, and even a few horses through the years.

I won't bore you with a long list of the pets that have gone over the Rainbow Bridge in my lifetime, but I do want to share some stories that I posted on my blogs over more recent years.

GOODBYE, MISS KITTY

One sad day, I had to do that thing that most pet owners dread. I had to have one of our kitties put to sleep. This was not the first animal I'd had to do this for, but it was the first after my husband and I had moved to our place in rural East Texas.

This was a stray that I rescued from a busy street in town because I couldn't stand the thought of her getting killed, and I just had a sense that she would if I left her. Not that we needed another cat. We already had three, all the products of someone dumping a pregnant cat along our county road, which was a favorite dumping ground for unwanted cats, dogs, kittens, and puppies. And this cat was pregnant for sure.

Miss Kitty, as we'd come to call her during the few weeks she lived with us, suddenly stopped eating one day, so I took her to the veterinarian. Turned out, she had feline leukemia and was so anemic the veterinarian was shocked that she was even still alive. She was also about two weeks shy of delivering what he guessed was her first litter of kittens.

The doctor said that Miss Kitty was so sick, treatment was not a viable option. Not news I wanted to hear, nor news he was particularly eager to share. In addition, he didn't think the kittens were still alive. He hadn't been able to detect movement, and, even if they were alive, they were probably infected.

So, we made the tough decision.

We'd only had Miss Kitty for about four weeks, but I'd really gotten attached in that short time. She was a sweet little gray and white tabby that purred every time I touched her and never offered to scratch or bite even when I was cleaning out the mites in her ears. I have scars from doing that with other cats.

Despite the fact that I knew this had to be done, I was still surprised at how emotional I got when the doctor gave the fatal injection. I cried as much for her as I had other pets that had been in my life much longer. I know we grieve for animals, even though there are some who think that is silly, but I really didn't expect the depth of grief I felt for this little cat.

In reflection, I see that this is just another example of what I've come to believe is true about grief. There are no rules. No timelines. No reasonable explanations for how it happens. It just is. The important thing is to acknowledge it and move through it.

ORCA AND JOHN

In addition to Miss Kitty, we had a number of other cats in the years that we lived out in the country in East Texas. At first, we just allowed the cats that wandered onto our property to live outside. We'd feed them and make sure they had water and a comfy place to sleep in the barn, but they couldn't come inside. We have family members who are allergic to cats so it had been many years since one had been allowed to cross our threshold.

Several years into our life out in the country, we noticed that the coyote population was growing in the area and coming closer to our place. That raised concerns about the safety of the cats, especially at night. We hated the thought that one of them would become coyote dinner, so we started bringing them in at night.

That wasn't an easy decision to make considering the allergies in the family, but visits to Grandma's Ranch had dwindled to only two or three a year, and I could clean really good before each visit. The cats would be closed up in the master bedroom and visitors were able to make it through the day.

One of the cats we had at that time was Orca, a black and white tuxedo cat. We called him our miracle cat because of what a tough life he had in his first three years. The fact that we had him for that long was in itself a bit of a miracle as out in the country the lifespan of a cat is much shorter than that of their city cousins. But we always tried to give them as much help as we could.

When Orca was just a kitten, he got into the engine of my husband's truck to take a nap and got caught up in the fan belt when my husband started the truck. Orca survived that, to the amazement of the farmer next door who came to help us get the cat out of the belt, as well as the veterinarian who repaired the broken leg.

After that mishap, Orca managed to avoid any more life-threatening scrapes for a little over two years. Then one Monday afternoon, he disappeared. Because he and his litter mate, John, would often stay out for a day or two, despite our best efforts, we didn't know that Orca was definitely gone until late Tuesday when he still had not come back to eat. He liked to be outside—preferring to use the sand in the yard instead of the litter box—plus there were all the moles and gophers and mice to hunt. But he didn't often miss the feeding times with the other cats, so we started to worry that he'd met up with a coyote or a car speeding down the road.

For three days we tried to keep the worry at bay and hold out a small hope that he might come back, but by Friday, we had to admit that probably wasn't going to happen.

That was a slam to our hearts.

Then late the following Sunday, Mother's Day, I was talking to one of my daughters on the phone. I'd just told her the sad tale of Orca's disappearance when I heard a mewing on the front porch. I looked out the window, paused a moment to make sure, then said, "Oh, my God. You'll never believe this. Orca's back."

"What a perfect Mother's Day present," my daughter said.

After hanging up, I went to open the front door, and Orca sauntered in—as best he could saunter dragging another broken leg—went right to his food dish and asked for supper. He ate, then went to take a nap on our bed, as if nothing had happened. My husband and I were in a state of shock for an hour or so, taking turns looking at him on the bed to make sure we weren't dreaming.

We weren't dreaming.

Somehow, Orca had managed to survive six days out in the wild and didn't even look too malnourished. We couldn't see any other injuries, either, and he didn't seem to be in much pain from the obviously mangled leg. He'd jumped up on the bed without a wince or a whimper, so we didn't do an emergency doctor visit, opting to take him to the animal clinic the next morning.

As it turned out, Orca had a nasty, splintered break below the knee and a dislocated knee, and we gulped when the veterinarian said how much it would cost a lot to repair all that. We briefly considered not repairing it, but then we figured if this cat could survive being caught up in a truck engine, being hit by another car, and then be out in the wild for six days with that injury, avoiding coyotes and other predatory animals, he deserved the other seven lives he had left.

That may not have been practical, but sometimes it feels good not to be practical.

John, who was sometimes called Big John after he outgrew his name, Little John, came from the same litter as Orca. Our neighbor had the mother, and when we decided we wanted another cat after losing the latest outside one that had disappeared, our neighbor talked us into taking two. They were the last kittens in the litter, and our neighbor was eager to find homes for them.

During the almost five years of his life, John didn't have

the accidents that Orca did, much to the relief of our hearts and our bank account, but one Friday night he disappeared. Then Orca disappeared for the last time late on Sunday of that same weekend. It's hard enough to lose one pet, but to lose two cats so closely together really slammed into our hearts. That's when we decided that we'd no longer have cats that went outside.

Currently, I have four cats who stay inside with me. These are cats that my husband and I got from a couple who rescued litters of kittens from the local animal shelter. They would hand-feed the kittens when the mother cat had died, and we were happy to be able to give the kittens a home when they were old enough to leave the special care.

POPPY

While I've primarily been a cat person, I've had a number of canine companions through the years, starting with Poochy, a little black dog we had when I was a kid, up to the dog I have now, Dusty. I won't go through the history of all the canine friends I've had, but I do want to share this blog post I wrote about one very special dog, Poppy, whose loss cut me deeply.

Poppy was my husband's dog first. I got her as an early birthday present for him one October because he'd been saying he'd like a Border Collie. Our neighbors had a great dog, Bear, and Carl thought it would be nice to have a dog like that, too. Poppy was a mix of Border Collie and Australian Shepard, but that was close enough.

MARYANN MILLER

Just before making the decision to move from the country to the city in 2017, I wrote this about Poppy. Instead of trying to paraphrase the older blog post, here it is in its entirety:

It's hard to believe, but it is four years to the day since my husband, Carl, died. Thoughts of him, and the life we shared here at Grandma's Ranch, have been poignant of late as I prepare to sell the property and move.

I wonder how my dog, Poppy, will fare in the city after the move. She has always been a country dog, with five acres to run on, so it will be quite an adjustment to only have a large back yard.

Poppy is now eleven years old, so I know there are not many years left that I will share with her. Her age is wearing her down, just as mine is reminding me that I am not thirty-nine, so I've decided to make whatever time she has left special. She is no longer banned from all people food. I give her a little bite now and then, and she is most happy about that.

Despite her eagerness to chase the ball and go walking with me, Poppy can no longer walk, or run, as far as she used to. So, I'm being careful on how many times I throw the ball, or how far I take her on the morning walk. It's great that I can leave her a good ways up my driveway and tell her to stay, so I can walk a little farther down the road. When I return, she's always where I left her, waiting for me to tell her what a good dog she is.

Because of her breeding, it's not surprising that Poppy is so smart. I know I will never have a dog as smart and as good as she is. She trained easily, and quickly, to basic commands and good manners, and there are times I swear she understands full sentences.

When I come back from the second leg of my morning walk, she sometimes greets me with her tennis ball nearby, which means she left her "stay" spot long enough to fetch it, just in case I might want to throw it once or twice. Ball chasing is limited now, and there are several things I say to end the play, "We're done." "That's all." "Just one more." "Poppy, I'm done."

No matter which phrase I use, she knows to stop where she is and lie down as there will be no more ball playing at the moment. She also understands, "I'm going in now." And will drop the ball and follow me into the house. I could still be standing halfway to the barn when I say that, so she's not just conditioned to respond when I step up to the back porch.

Poppy managed to live almost two more years after I wrote that blog post, making the move to the city with me in January 2018, only to get a brain tumor a few weeks later. After numerous trips to the veterinarian for testing and exams, it became clear there was no alternative other than the one all pet owners hate to face. I made the tough decision to have her put down. She'd gone downhill fast, and only a few weeks after the first symptoms appeared, she could barely walk in the house or around the backyard. She started listing to one side, stumbling and losing her balance, and it was obvious things were not going well for her.

That was probably the most significant, and difficult, pet loss of my life. Perhaps because of Poppy's connection to my husband, and perhaps because it was just one more loss piled onto so many in recent years; my father, my husband, my mother, my place in the country, my horse and other animals, and now this wonderful dog. No other dog will have my heart like Poppy did.

MARYANN MILLER

THE IMPORTANCE OF HAVING NO REGRETS AT THE END OF LIFE

As we grow older and start looking at that time when we must "go gently into that goodnight" as Dylan Thomas wrote, that's when we assess what we've done, or not done, and figure out how gentle that will be for us. In all of the death journeys I was privileged to share with patients and families, the ones that had fewer regrets were the easiest.

While I understood that from a clinical standpoint, the lesson didn't come home to me until a few years later, when I was no longer working as a chaplain. The following is a blog post I wrote a few years after my husband and I moved back to Texas.

As I was clearing brush from my back pasture today, I reflected on how I almost didn't follow my dream of having acreage and playing farmer.

When my husband and I were preparing to move back to Texas after our stint in Nebraska, we knew it would probably be our last move, and we wanted to make sure it would be a home that we would be happy in the rest of our lives. For my husband, that didn't mean much beyond a house with a large master bedroom and a walk-in shower in the bathroom. Other than that, he didn't care.

On the other hand, I cared a lot. I wanted a house with a large country kitchen, some character, and a nice room for my office where I would write my books. And, in my heart of hearts, I wanted to live in the country on a few acres where I might be able to have a horse. Yet, I wasn't even sure if I should attempt to have that because my husband's health was not good, and I thought we should settle for a nice house in a small town.

When I told one of the chaplains I worked with what I was considering versus what I really wanted, she asked me, "Why are you settling, Maryann?"

"I'm not settling. I'm being practical."

"But what if you regret not following your heart?"

She countered my every argument, finally ending with, "What will it matter if you only get to live your dream for a few years before circumstances force another move? Is giving up really what you want to do?"

I considered what she said and it all made sense. I didn't want to end up on my death bed playing that sad old "what if" game.

Buoyed with her advice, I told my husband that I was going to look at acreage the next time we went house-hunting in Texas. I thought he might object, but bless his heart, he didn't. Of course, he'd picked all the homes we'd lived in previously and had told me this selection was mine, so he really couldn't object.

After much searching that must have driven our realtor into despair as to whether there would ever be a place that would satisfy me, perhaps making her consider looking for another profession, we found our perfect house. Well, maybe not perfect, but close to it, and it came with a walk-in shower, large master bedroom, large kitchen, and almost seven acres.

Shortly after moving in, we had a back and front pasture fenced in, and I got my horse, followed closely by two goats.

Our little city dog, Misha, adapted well to country living, rarely leaving the property, but then it was so much bigger than the small back yard she'd been accustomed to, and she lived several years there before crossing over the Rainbow Bridge.

Our next-door neighbors, as in about two acres to the north, were country folks from way back, and they helped this greenhorn learn a lot about taking care of animals and acreage and gardens. They were so kind and never, okay maybe a couple of times, laughed when I came over with a problem that seemed so simple to them. I learned a lot from them, and our friendship reminded me of why I'd always appreciated and respected farmers for their love of the land.

My husband and I lived out there in the country together for nearly fifteen years before he died from a massive heart attack. I managed to stay five more years, living alone, except for my critters, until my health issues forced a move to a small city, closer to kids and specialists.

I miss my husband, and I miss that beautiful place we had that was so peaceful. He once said that the Piney Woods of East Texas was the most pastoral place he'd ever been in.

I agree. It was a place of quiet beauty, where one couldn't help but feel close to God, and every day I thanked Him for the wisdom of my chaplain friend, as well as the many blessings of "Grandma's Ranch."

When death comes knocking, I'll have few regrets.

GIFTS FROM OTHERS

The following is a post I wrote in 2012. This was a year before my husband died. Again, I share the post as originally written:

Today a dear friend called to tell me her husband died yesterday. I knew the time was close. Jan had called last month to tell me Dave was terminal and in hospice care. He was at home, on the family farm that they had taken over when his parents retired from farming, and he was ready to take that step into the other place. He believed that other place is heaven and so do I. He told Jan that he'd a glimpse of it when he almost died the previous month.

My friend and I spent an hour on the phone today sharing about Dave and all the good times we had as couples when my husband and I would visit their little corner of the world in South Dakota. Dave had an incredible sense of humor, and Jan said she still has the joke book he compiled years ago. She said it is filed in the filing cabinet under "J". Of course it is.

The only thing that wasn't satisfying about the call was having to end it by both of us acknowledging that I wouldn't be able to go up there for Dave's funeral. My husband's health was such that I couldn't get away. Jan, being the special friend that she is, told me that was okay. I'd been there with her other times when she needed me, especially through the death of her father and mother.

One of the many things I learned from her and her family was how to accept what life throws at you. I think farmers have an insight about that beyond what some of the rest of us have. It's like on one hand there's all the sadness and grief that comes with losing someone you love, but on another plane is that realization that this is all so natural and so right. There is life and there is death. Period.

Jan and I have been friends since we were eleven years old, and she and her family have been such an important part of my life. I lived with them for a few years after I graduated from high school, and then later Jan moved away and so did I. We stayed in touch - she from South Dakota and me from Texas - but I didn't see her for nineteen years. The first time I made a trip north from Texas, it was like those nineteen years melted away.

When my husband and I moved from Texas to Omaha NE, that closer proximity allowed us to go visit Jan and Dave several times a year for weekends. That was always in the spring, summer, or fall, and only once in the winter when we buried Jan's mother just before a blizzard hit. Those were very special years, a time during which I really got to know and appreciate Dave, a man I'd only met briefly before. He was a Navy veteran of the Vietnam war and had some of the problems those who have seen combat carry like excess baggage, but he was also kind and generous and loyal to his family and friends.

So today Jan and I cried a bit together and then shared more memories of Dave. Before we ended the call, she asked me what I was doing today. I told her I was getting ready to go to the Comedy Show at the art center. She chuckled, "Dave would like that."

Yeah, I think he would. Despite the great burden he carried because of his war experience, he did enjoy a good joke.

MOM MILLER'S GIFT

During the years we lived in Nebraska, we always took two weeks or a little more to go back to Texas for the Christmas and New Year's holidays. Spending those special times with our kids was important to us, so we always looked forward to the visits, and that year was no exception.

We'd just arrived at our son's house when we got a call that my husband's mother had died. That was December 18, 2001. We flew to Michigan the next day for the funeral that took place a couple of days later, and managed to get back to Texas late on the 23rd.

This is a blog post I wrote a few years later as part of the series on grief.

There is no good time to lose someone you love, but close to holidays, especially the winter holidays of Christmas, Chanukah, and Kwanza, grief has a sharper edge. Excitement is in the air like electricity as people bustle around preparing for visits by relatives and warm, family times; and for some there is a huge hole in the gathering.

People deal with that fact of life and death in different ways, but I never realized how many reactions there are until I started facilitating grief support groups. When grieving a loss, some people abandon all normal traditions, finding it too difficult to consider the usual holiday dinner with someone missing. Others don't have the emotional energy to decorate or shop. The one thing to remember is that whatever a grieving family decides to do, that's okay.

Often, we're pressured by some perceived convention of

what is the "proper" thing to do, and the truth is, there is no one-size-fits-all way to behave. For us, the year that Mom Miller died just before Christmas, we all put on a smiling face and carried on with the normal family traditions. Not because we thought we had to, but because we knew that was the best way to honor her. We soothed our aching hearts with the knowledge that she had lived a long, wonderful life, and she had been more than ready to go to heaven for ten years. On Christmas day, we smiled a bittersweet smile when we raised a toast to her at dinner.

Mom really loved a party.

It wasn't the best Christmas we ever had, but it worked because we decided how to react to our grief instead of letting the grief control us. And that little bit of control is a key element to surviving the holidays while grieving. We can't control the fates, or nature, or whatever it is that brings the devastation of death, but we can control what happens next. We can do whatever it takes to get through. Some people go off on a trip, away from a home that seems so empty, yet holds so many memories. Many people abandon the traditional family dinner and go to a restaurant. Some families forgo gifts and donate to a charity in memory of the person they lost.

Whatever a person does, it's important to remember that even with the best of plans, the grief can surge and blindside you without notice. According to Laura Slap-Shelton, Psy.D., "This is because our best and worst memories are often generated in the crucible of holiday celebration. As the holidays come upon us, we are both unconsciously and consciously reminded of our lost loved one."

Mom Miller's final gift to us was quite a surprise. Despite

her best efforts to spend all her money before she died, there was a small inheritance for each of her four children. It wasn't a huge amount, but enough for us to take a road trip from Texas to Michigan. We also decided that we'd use part of that little windfall to take my mother to Mackinaw Island for lunch at the Grand Hotel.

My mother, sister, and I had made several trips to the island in years past, and Mother would sit outside the hotel, often saying how much she wished she could afford to go inside. At the time, our meager vacation funds would never even cover the admission charge for a tour of the hotel grounds.

So, I'd talked my husband into splurging on lunch for my mother, my sister, and the two of us. I told him it would be one of the finest gifts we could give my mother, and he agreed.

No cars are allowed on the island, except for security vehicles, so we took a carriage ride from the ferry landing to the hotel. There, we were seated at an exquisitely set table with fine linen, silver and crystal, and Mother had her own waiter who seated her and put a napkin on her lap. I was thrilled for my mother, who was actually flirting with her waiter and loving every moment of being treated like royalty, but I couldn't help but think of how Mom Miller would have enjoyed the afternoon. That brought a warmth of tears to my eyes, and I asked everyone if we could lift a glass to toast Mom Miller and thank her for the gift of this special day.

There was no objection.

As I've learned with subsequent losses, it takes time for the pain of the grief to diminish to a point that every holiday and special occasion is not measured against the loss, but eventually the ache subsides to a tolerable level. There will never be another Christmas that I don't think of Mom Miller, and all the others who have gone before me, but today it hurts a little less.

LOSS OF HEALTH

When serious illness strikes, it brings with it so many challenges, and it's important to recognize the grieving process that is part of what is happening. We may lose strength and mobility. No more exercising. Or shopping. Or playing with the kids. There is a great deal of anxiety and fear. Will we ever be okay again? Are we looking into that dark hole that is ahead of us all?

The year that I was recovering from kidney surgery, or not recovering so well as it turned out, severe pain and some muscle weakness brought significant limitations. In addition to not being able to sit very long at my computer to work, or have the strength to play with my kids, or exercise, I was also not able to do any gardening. Not that I had a huge garden at our house in a suburb of Dallas, but I did always have flowers in the two front flowerbeds. It pained my heart that I wasn't able to be out digging in the dirt, and I processed that heartache in an article:

Pretty little flowers all in a row.

Not that year.

That year a few scraggly weeds lived in the spots usually reserved for the pansies that thrived early in the Texas growing season. Normally, when the sun burned too hot, the pansies would be replaced with petunias, then later with periwinkles. Those hardy little flowers can thumb their noses at the worst heat thrown at them.

Attending to this ritual of planting has always been an important part of my existence. Some days I'd rather be out digging in the dirt than doing almost anything else. The process feeds me deep inside in a way that defies articulation. But those who share this passion understand.

When it was time to plant the pansies that year, I was in the hospital after a complicated kidney surgery. The weeks recuperating at home ate up the rest of early spring when cool nights and mild days nurtured the 'people' flowers and let them smile to greet a new day.

My heart ached when I was strong enough to walk out to the front porch and sit on the swing. The empty flower beds looked so lost and forgotten, and I yearned to dig my hands into the dirt. I thought of asking my husband to plant something, just a geranium or two for a splash of color, but resisted the urge on two counts. He had enough to do with taking care of the kids, the house, and his job. Plus, it wasn't the flowers I missed so much as the process. I could wait a few more weeks and still have plenty of growing season left. It lasts forever in Texas.

Petunia season came and went, and still the flowerbeds stood empty.

I'd had a bit of a set-back in my recovery. Some nerves had been damaged during the hours-long surgery and the pain was still incredibly severe. That forced another trip to the hospital to see if anything could be done.

By the time I got home again, we were well into periwinkle season and my flowerbeds had grown lush with weeds. My instinct was to lean forward in the swing and pluck out a clump of clover, but the look from my husband, rich with unsaid words, stilled the impulse.

I'm sure he meant well. Like so many spouses standing on the outside he felt so helpless in the face of my pain and limitations. He only wanted to protect me. But my heart yearned to be digging in the dirt. It was a deep and powerful ache that wouldn't go away.

During my next visit to the doctor, I asked if he thought it would be okay to do a bit of gardening. "I'll be careful," I said. "And I just feel this great need."

The man could have posed for a Norman Rockwell painting as he sat on his little black stool with one finger tapping his cheek. Then he spoke. "Personally, I think there's something very healing about dirt. Although I don't recommend eating it."

He paused to acknowledge the smile with timing so perfect he could've been on the comedy circuit. "But I do recommend filling your hands with it. Smell it. Work it. Let it fall through your fingers. It won't cure you, but it won't hurt, either. And maybe it will make you feel better where it matters."

Several hours later I knelt on the grass. I ignored the pain that ran down my side and into my leg and leaned close to the dirt. The trowel felt good in my hand as I loosened a small section of the flowerbed. Then I picked up clumps of earth and crumbled them, letting the rich black dirt stream through my fingers. I reveled in the cool dampness; the pungent aroma. Then I dug a hole big enough to hold a single Marigold.

"Ah," my heart said. "Just what you needed."

Now, many years later, I'm challenged by trigeminal neuralgia, a lingering gift from Ramsay Hunt Syndrome, as well as arthritis and other signs of aging. These things limit me, much the way the complications of that surgery did, and I have

MOVING

The following blog post is one I wrote almost three years ago. Like others I've been sharing, I thought it best to include it verbatim:

As someone who resists even rearranging the furniture in a room, imagine how hard it is for me to deal with a major change.

I am also a person who puts down deep roots in a place, so it is hard for me to pull them up and go to another city or state. The heel marks between Dallas and Omaha, NE when my husband's job took us there, was not just because I was reluctant to leave my kids. I was reluctant to leave my house, my friends, my church, my comfort zone and go to a strange new place.

The move from Omaha back to Texas was tough on many levels, but still not quite as hard, as I was coming back closer to my kids. Plus, I was going to live my childhood dream of a place in the country and having my very own horse in my very own back pasture. That horse would be there to greet me in the morning with a nicker when I went out with my first cup of coffee.

Banjo did say a cheery hello every morning for the past fifteen years, but it was not always a greeting of affection. More often, it was a reminder that I needed to go to the barn and get his hay. He was highly motivated by food.

Now Banjo is gone, as are all my other big animals. A very nice man bought Banjo, and took the sheep, Marie, who was Banjo's only pasture mate after we lost our goat. They will both have a good home with that man for the rest of their lives. He promised they wouldn't end up at market, and a farmer's word is as good as gold in the country. So even though I cried when they left, and still get a lump in my throat when I go outside, that grief is tempered with the knowledge that they will be well taken care of.

Even so, it was so hard to go outside and see that empty pasture.

The animals are gone because I made the difficult decision a few weeks ago to sell my property and move to the Dallas area to be closer to my kids - and closer to doctors that I need to see there.

This has all been very hard emotionally as I waver between thinking about how much I will miss this place in the country, my animals, and my wonderful community of friends in Winnsboro, and believing that this is the right thing to do. It IS the right thing to do, and the way some things have fallen into place so quickly, only affirms that for me.

Still, the change is hard, and knowing that I am not the only one who struggles with change, I did some Internet browsing and happened upon this article at the Harvard Business Review: Ten Reasons People Resist Change by Rosabeth Moss Kanter. She's a professor at Harvard Business School and chair and director of the Harvard Advanced Leadership Initiative.

The article addresses change in the workplace, but many of the points can be applied to any kind of change.

Loss of control

Uncertainty

Everything is different

More work

Loss of face

That last one made me pause a moment to see how it applied to my situation. Kanter explained that:

"By definition, change is a departure from the past. Those people associated with the last version — the one that didn't work, or the one that's being superseded — are likely to be defensive about it... Leaders can help people maintain dignity by celebrating those elements of the past that are worth honoring, and making it clear that the world has changed. That makes it easier to let go and move on.

When I move from this place, it will be a departure from the past. My face will no longer be the face of a country woman or Theatre Director at the Winnsboro Center for the Arts. Everything will be different and there is a great deal of uncertainty about what my new face(s) will be.

I know a lot about the importance of rituals in dealing with tough emotional situations. Most of that I learned when

MARYANN MILLER

I put on a new face as a hospital chaplain in Omaha after leaving my old face as a journalist and PR consultant in Dallas those many years ago. But if I had not made that move, I would not have experienced the personal growth I went through during my Clinical Pastoral Education, as well as the blessings of working in a hospital, ministering to the sick. Nor would I have met so many friends in two writers' groups, most of whom still stay in contact with me.

So, I'll perform some good-bye rituals when I'm leaving my place and try my best to focus on the future and what adventures will await me down the road.

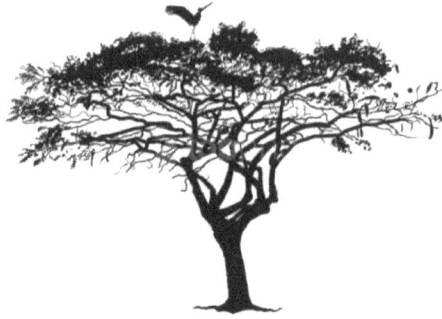

MY OWN GRIEF JOURNEY

We experience all kinds of losses in our life, big and small, and the grieving can be most difficult when deaths, and other life-changing events, pile one upon the other very quickly, like leaves falling from the trees in Autumn. That was true for me over a relatively short period of years when my father died, then my husband died, followed by my mother, and then one of my sisters. I remember that after my husband died, I prayed very hard that I could have at least a year before my mother would follow him. Despite the differences in ages, 76 for him and 92 for her, they were both in failing health at the same time, and I was never sure if I could survive losing them both close together. I needed time to recover from one before another loss hit.

I had six months.

My husband died in September 2013. Mother died March 2014.

Of all of these deaths, my husband's had the most impact,

and, even though I thought I was preparing myself over the years that he suffered with diabetes, as well as heart and lung problems, I wasn't prepared at all.

My husband had his first major heart attack while we still lived in Omaha, that resulted in a five-way heart bypass. During the weeks and months following that surgery, I learned another big lesson about grieving and a few things about myself.

While I was so good at helping others, I fell short at helping myself, and I felt so inadequate when it came to helping my husband. He was angry. A lot. He took it out on nurses when he was in the hospital. He took it out on dieticians who tried to help him understand the importance of adopting a healthier way of eating, and he took it out on me when he had nobody else to rail at.

The chaplain on our team that worked in the cardiac unit explained some of what happens when a person has a heart attack, and how the physical is connected to the emotional. A physical broken heart often reflects an emotional broken heart. Not always in the romantic sense, but following some personal devastation of another sort.

I could attest to that. Carl had been laid off from several jobs in the previous seven years. The first a real kick in the gut after he'd worked at a company for twenty-three years. He was forty-nine at the time and soon discovered that age discrimination is alive and well. He was unable to land another full-time job, and we struggled to stay afloat financially, almost losing our house at one point. He worked a few consulting jobs in different states, finally going to Nebraska with the promise of a full-time job with a consulting firm, only to lose that job six months after bringing me up from Texas.

In addition to the job loss, Carl had been kicked in the heart when a difficult situation had developed in our church in Texas, creating extreme hard feeling in a lot of parishioners. Through no fault of his own, Carl was the brunt of people expressing many of those feelings, ultimately leading to him voluntarily step back from ministry for a year when he realized it wasn't good for the parish or for him to stay. Perhaps the divisions among the people would heal if he was not there.

It's no wonder the poor man had a heart attack. His heart was in such pain, but he didn't want to talk about it. In addition to refusing to talk to the dietician, he wanted no part of seeing that chaplain or joining the support group for patients who had had heart surgery.

What he did was go home and retreat, like a bear going into a cave every winter, and there were many days I was afraid to poke that bear.

Luckily, that first round of depression only lasted a few months. When he was able to be active again, serving the church as a deacon in our new parish in Omaha, he also volunteered to be the chaplain for the local St. Vincent DePaul organization that serves the poor in a community. That work brought some joy into his eyes, and I was pleased that the darkness had been pulled back for a time.

I could also see that when we went back to Texas every year for our extended holiday visit with our kids and grandkids, he'd be incredibly happy and animated. It soon became clear that we should probably pack up and go home. At that point, I didn't know how many years Carl had left before his heart gave up for the last time, but I wanted those years to be spent with all the people that he loved.

Plus, he hated the snow.

So, that's what precipitated our move to East Texas.

Fast forward many years and through many heart-related, or diabetes related, problems to Thursday, September 5, 2013. Carl and I had a leisurely breakfast, during which we had one of the best talks we'd had in some time, and he left to do his volunteer stint at the Winnsboro Center For the Arts. Thursdays were his days to man the desk and answer the phone, and this was his first day back after having a minor heart attack almost a month earlier, that landed him in the hospital for several days.

But he was home now, and feeling better than he had in quite a while, so neither of us even anticipated that this was our last morning together. Shortly after opening the art center, he had a massive heart attack and was rushed to the hospital after friends found him down on the floor.

Even after all these years, some details are still clear in my mind. What I was doing when my friend called to tell me that Carl was at the hospital. What I said to her, which was a litany of cuss words. Calling a neighbor to come over and take care of my horse who was tied out in the yard for mowing duty. Calling one of my daughters. Telling her I couldn't call the other kids. Would she?

Yes.

Somehow, I sensed the worst.

Frantically trying to decide if I should change from my farmer clothes to my going-to-town clothes.

My friends coming to drive me to the hospital. They didn't want me to drive. I think they knew.

Nerves jangling the whole way there.

Being slammed with the news.

Tears.

Hugs.

Prayers.

Then, nothing.

I don't remember coming home. I think my friend drove me. None of my kids were there yet, so I was alone, but this "alone" was so different from the alone when Carl was at the store. Or at the art center. Or at church for a meeting with other clergy. This "alone" was going to be forever.

As I write this today, I realize that I never actually put those words to the situation before—alone forever. I never fully accepted the reality that I was singular now. Not a half of a couple. Just one person.

Alone forever.

Wow! Why did it take so long for me to acknowledge that? Perhaps because denial can be an ongoing part of dealing with loss. Not the denial that he was gone, but the inability to look at that horrible reality of "alone" with open eyes and an open heart.

I found the following in my grief journal, written just five months after Carl died. "Normally one looks at a new chapter in her life as an adventure. I think back on all the new chapters that my life wrote for me in the years after I married, and so many were challenges, yet positive. It is so hard to begin another new chapter when someone is missing from the story. I know that is one of the things that has been holding me captive. I don't want to do this. I don't want a life without Carl."

Sometimes we take giant steps through the grieving process and other times baby steps. Thank goodness there is no timeline for any of this. And as one friend of mine put it after her husband died, "Grief doesn't ever really end – it just changes."

While working at the hospital and facilitating those grief support groups, I learned that it is imperative to keep taking those steps. It's also important, as part of a healthy grieving process, to work toward not focusing so much on what is lost, but looking at what we have.

So, I try to look at all the good things we had together for all those years.

In addition to the wonderful family that Carl and I had, and all the kids and grandkids that filled our home and our lives with joy, I had that one last good day with him.

We'd just celebrated our forty-eighth wedding anniversary and were so hoping we would make it to fifty. Since his health had been so fragile for a year or more, we both knew that was a real long-shot, but we hoped nonetheless. That's what people do, right? You don't just stop and wait for that final moment.

Now, today, I look back at that awful September day in 2013, and I try to take comfort in the fact that we had a little over two weeks of really good days from the time he came home from the hospital August 19 and the day he died. He felt better than he had in months, and that dark mood that had made him so depressed had lifted. He smiled. It was like the sun coming out from a dark cloud. You know. That dazzling brightness that almost takes your breath away.

Today, I can smile through my tears, but that doesn't mean I don't miss him. Or I'm "over it." We never get over losing a partner, or anyone in our lives for that matter. It's just that the pain of missing him isn't with me 24/7 anymore. Slowly, as months and years march on, we adjust to the shift in our lives and have more days of no pain of grief that string together to form … maybe a whole week.

I think that's why his sudden death that Thursday morning was such a shock. I had dared to hope that those good days we were having would stretch into good weeks, then good months, and maybe a few more good years.

MY FATHER

The fun of April First and all the April Fool jokes lost its appeal for me some years ago when my father died on that day. I can still remember my sister's exact words when she called to tell me the news. "This isn't an April Fool's Day joke, Maryann. Wanted to be sure you knew that before I tell you that Daddy died."

She didn't really have to tell me it wasn't a joke. I could tell by the tremor in her voice it was something serious. Daddy had been in a nursing home for a few weeks following a stroke, and I had just been down to Houston to see him. Before I left to go back home, he'd been showing some improvement, and we all thought he would get better, so his death was a bit of a shock to us all.

Since then, I've had a hard time entering into the fun of April First and all the jokes.

In 2018, Easter fell on April first, and brought with it thoughts of my father. We who are Christian and celebrate Easter and the Resurrection of Jesus, believe that we all share in that Resurrection when we've lived a good and honorable life.

My father did just that. He wasn't in a church pew on Sundays, although he did attend important milestones in my religious journey, but most of all, he lived that good and honorable life. Not perfect, but good, and he instilled in me, and my siblings, a sense of integrity, compassion, a strong work ethic, and loyalty to family and friends.

I was honored when my sisters and brothers asked me to speak at the funeral, and here are just a few of the things I shared that day:

It was my father who told me so many years ago that it is not so foolish to pursue a dream.

It was my father who told me that I should make choices in my life according to what would make me happy, even if the world doesn't approve of my choices.

It was my father who told me to give an honest day's work for an honest day's wage.

It was my father who told me to consider any stranger a potential new friend.

It was my father who told me that it's not what you are that's important, but who you are.

And above all, it was my father who told me that while he didn't have much to show for his life; no big house, no fancy car, no grand retirement spot where he could spend his social security in luxury, he had us, his children, to stand as monuments of accomplishment. He considered it time well spent.

It's no surprise then, that family is my greatest treasure.

MY MOTHER

My mother, Evelyn, had a heart attack on March 24, 2014, and she died on March 28. I was able to get to Michigan the Wednesday prior, so I had two days to say my final goodbye, even though my heart was not ready to do that yet. On Thursday, she had that bloom that people often get before they are going to die. Mother was sitting up, looking good, enjoying the company, and for a little while we forgot that she was probably not going to survive the heart attack and the flu that had settled in on top of that.

It was a very blessed day. The kind of day that all families should have when they are about to lose someone so dear to them, especially if they can make the most of it, and we did. We told stories, we sang songs, and all of the people who loved her dearly came by with their hugs and kisses and memories.

Friday morning, it was obvious that our hopes were not going to come true, and Mother passed early that afternoon.

The following Wednesday, April 2, two of my kids, Mike and Dany, helped me sing Mother to Heaven. That was a bit unusual, I know, but the church that she was connected to didn't have their music ministers available. None of us in the family thought that Mother should have a funeral without music, so my niece borrowed two guitars from friends—one for me and one for Dany—and Mike added his beautiful voice to the make-shift choir. The hymns were ones that I remembered my mother particularly liking from when I'd sat in pews with her at Mass, and we sang and played through many tears during that bittersweet experience.

My sister and I planned the funeral service, making sure that all of the grandchildren would have a role of some kind, as that is so important in saying goodbye. Some were readers. Some were pall bearers. Some were Eucharistic Ministers. Some brought up the gifts at offertory, and one of my daughters, Anjanette, read a story she had written, "Evelyn and the Blue Bunny".

Mother had introduced me to the book *Bunny Blue* when I was a child, and the tattered copy of that children's book was one of the few I saved into adulthood. I then shared it with my kids, and then it was passed on to grandkids. It is such a wonderful story that we all have loved, and I'm sure my mother was smiling to hear her granddaughter read her story.

While there were many blessed moments during that time, my heart was still very heavy, bearing the weight of the loss. Not only did I miss my mother, and her letters that always included a drawing of some sort, I had the stark realization that with her and my father gone, there was nobody ahead of me anymore.

MY SISTER

As the years march on, it's inevitable that we will not only lose parents, as part of the natural course of life, but our older siblings will also go before us. The following is the eulogy that my brothers and sisters asked me to deliver when our oldest sister died. Different members of the family spoke of her as mother and grandmother, and a few friends shared what their friendship meant. I spoke as a sister:

Rosanne was my oldest sister, the oldest of six siblings. There were times it was hard for me to remember that there were only eight years between Rosanne and me. She always seemed to be the one adult among us kids, and then there was the space that separated us. My parents divorced when I was five, and my father married Rosanne's mother, when I was seven. When they married, there were her kids, his kids, and eventually their kids, two of each, and it took a while to stir that mix and end up with a family, but we managed to do that.

Rosanne married young and moved out of the home, so my earliest memories of her are when she would come by with Kathryn as a baby on the weekends that Juanita and I spent at the house. It was always busy and chaotic at the house on those weekends, but I do remember being so impressed with how grown up Rosanne was compared to the rest of us kids, and I was always a bit in awe of this adult sister.

One special time I remember from those early years, was a day when I was visiting her at her house. I think it was not long after Charlie was born. I was older then, and she treated me almost like a girlfriend her own age. We had lunch and she talked about her kids and the new home, and I recall how content she looked, so obviously happy to have a home of her own and a family. It seemed like life was going to be so good. And I remember thinking I would like that someday. I would like a home and a family and to be as happy as Rosanne seemed to be that day.

Even though her life wasn't always so happy, there is no doubt she continued to love family, especially her kids, and would do anything to keep them together and give them the best life possible.

Another memory that comes to mind is the time she drove me, Juanita, and Loreen down to West Virginia for Grandma Van Gilder's funeral. I don't remember for sure where we stayed down there, but it was a room with bunk beds. One night all four of us went out to a club with our cousin Kenny and got a little tipsy… okay a lot tipsy. Kenny loved to take us out for an evening of drink and frivolity, and we were always ready for a little frivolity. When we got back to the house, Nita and Loreen and I were all silly and giggly, and we kept Rosanne awake most of the night. She loved to tell that story on us, laughing as she recounted how Nita and I would lean from the top bunk to talk to her and she would tell us to "shut up and go to sleep."

I loved to hear her tell that story, as the telling was always tinged with so much love underneath the layer of mock frustration.

In recent years, I have started to recognize, and deeply appreciate, the great gifts that certain strong women have been in my life, and Rosanne was certainly one of those strong

THE MANY FACES OF GRIEF

women. When I think of all the challenges she overcame throughout her life, I stand in awe again. She endured losses that no parent should have to suffer and had so many physical challenges throughout the years, and yet she just kept on keeping on. Right until the end she was willing to fight one more battle before she finally said, "Okay it's time."

That iron will that gave her the strength to endure, to battle cancer, to endure even more physical and emotional pain was the same iron will that sometimes put us at odds. Often her kind heart was masked in a brusque manner that had her come across as harsh. But that was just her way. She didn't suffer fools easily and she never held back an opinion. There were times she scared me off with her manner and her harsh words but her intent was never to wound. Something with just bubble up inside her and had to come out. But isn't that the way all families operate? We don't always agree. We have harsh words. We hurt each other, but we get over it.

I had a lot of getting over it through the years with Rosanne, and the rocky patches were as much my fault as hers. I am so glad that I was finally able to admit that to her and reconcile a long time ago. Now, looking back over our life and our relationship, I realize that in many ways she was a better sister then I ever was. She was the first one to say why can't we just be sisters and not step-sisters. She was willing to forgive me for the hurts I had caused her and say let's move on.

And so we did.

From that point on we were able to be closer as sisters, and her enthusiasm for my writing was very special to me. She always asked about what I was working on, read my books and came to celebrate with me when I won awards. A year ago this past April, she came to Austin for one of those events, and I was so honored that she made that effort. Knowing how much pain she was in with her back problems, I didn't expect her to come, and I know the trip was not easy for her or for Wally. Still they came to support me, and I will always be grateful for that.

So as I say goodbye to my sister, not my step-sister, I will always treasure those good moments and let the not-so-good moments fade from my memory.

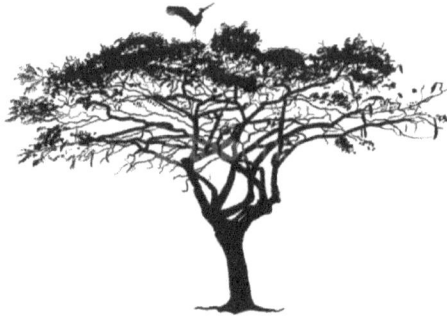

COMING OUT OF THE CLOUD
OF GRIEF

I t's taken most of two years I've lived in my new home in a new city to deal with the accumulation of grief from all those losses, and on clear days, I realized that I'm slowly recovering. I'm able to think about my husband without this great clutch of pain around my heart. When I think about my mother and my father and my sister, it's not always with the urge to cry with every memory.

What hasn't become easier, is coming to terms with the loss of my place out in the country and the critters I had there. In the fifteen years that I had Grandma's Ranch, my horse and goats became such an integral part of my being that my being still feels the pull to be there. I yearn for the blessed quiet, the beautiful scenery, the plethora of wildflowers that would dot the meadows and roadways with bold colors, and the animals that would help me greet each new day.

Here in the city there is none of that.

Still, I know that in order to be happier, I need to stop lamenting what is lost and focus on the joy that can be found here.

The same goes for what aging is taking away from me.

I am not growing old gracefully.

It was hard for me to admit that to myself the first time the thought flitted through my mind, and I had to say it a lot of times before I was able to bring it to this page. Perhaps growing older would have been easier without some of the significant health issues that have plagued me. I don't know, but I do know it was easier to look ahead to the golden years with eagerness when I was in my fifties and even sixties. A time when I was strong and active and healthy.

Many of the people in my extended family who lived well into their eighties and nineties were people who were very strong, like my grandmother. And I always thought I would be like them. Living "well" into my eighties and nineties and growing old gracefully.

Grandma Emma, who was my father's mother, marked her one hundredth birthday, plus two. Until a broken hip sent her to her bed, she was always working in her garden on the hillside behind her house. When she was inside, she kept busy baking and cooking quilting and hooking rugs. When I was there visiting, I never saw her sit down unless she was doing the handwork.

Many people in the family have often said how much I remind them of Grandma Emma. That was especially true when I was still living out in the country. While I didn't have a huge garden on a hillside behind my house, I did have a small garden, and I had a few acres to mow and keep clear of brush, as well as the animals to take care of every day. Those chores kept me active and strong and happy.

That activity came to a screeching halt when the trigeminal neuralgia I have caused so much pain that I just couldn't keep on keeping on. When that happened, I noticed how quickly my older body succumbed to new problems caused by not working hard and not being as active as I used to be.

~*~

My father used to say that any day you wake up on the grassy side of the dirt is a good day, and that is so true, but I also remember my mother-in-law saying how much old age sucked. She made that comment when health challenges had forced her to move from her apartment, where she'd been independent, to a nursing home. When we visited her in the facility, she often said she wished she could have died at home. I think most of us have a similar wish. If only we could choose the day and time without having to take our own lives and put that burden on our family, but we don't have a choice of when and where we will depart this earth, nor how difficult the last years will be.

Thinking about those last years, I recall a presentation that I attended as part of my CPE training. "Linda," one of the medical social workers, whose specialty was geriatrics, took us through the passages of life that most people experience. She started off the talk by introducing us to a fictional young married couple who bought their first house with three bedrooms and soon filled it up with furniture and children and all the things that make a house a home.

Then Linda took us forward to when that same couple grew older. The children married and moved away, and the house became too large for just two people. So, they sold the house and moved into a small apartment with just two bedrooms; one for them and one for the children when they came to visit. About ten years later, the couple's health started to deteriorate so they moved into an assisted living facility.

Each of those moves necessitated selling, or giving away, most of their furniture, as well as some prized possessions they no longer had room for.

A little more each time.

Then the husband died and the woman fell and broke her hip. She could no longer take care of herself and live alone, even in assisted living, so she ended up in a nursing home. The few cherished possessions that the couple had taken with them to the assisted living apartment had to be relinquished, and the old woman took just a shoebox full of special things with her to the nursing home.

That was a very poignant story and it really touched my heart when I heard it, but back then when I was in my fifties, I couldn't relate to the various stages that the couple went through. At the time, my husband and I were living in a small rental house, but we still had our bigger house in Texas, where we'd raised our kids. We still had most of our possessions, even though most of them were in boxes in the basement of the rental house. So, we had yet to feel that first major loss when one has to give up things that are family treasures and have so much sentimental value.

Now I'm beginning to internalize that couple's story.

THE MANY FACES OF GRIEF

While I am still far from being at the point of needing to put just a few things in a shoebox to take to a nursing home, my last move that brought me here to the city necessitated quite a bit of downsizing.

~*~

Like my mother-in-law said, I hope I die before I have to pack a shoebox. But if that doesn't happen, I'll try to be like a lady that I met a few years ago when I was doing a feature story about a new assisted living facility in the little town where I used to live. The lady had just come in to sign admittance papers and she was sitting in the lounge area. I sat down next to her and couldn't help but notice how happy she looked.

I thought maybe she'd come to meet a friend for lunch, but she quickly told me that she'd just become a resident. When I asked if it had been hard to make that decision, she acknowledged that it was, but then she smiled and said, "Still, I'm happy."

It was hard for me to understand how somebody could say that about such an abrupt change from what was known and loved to this new normal. She laughed and said, "We can choose to be unhappy or we can choose to be happy. Every day, I choose to be happy." What a great reminder of the truth that we have no control over the circumstances of our life, good or bad, but we have control over how we respond to those circumstances.

While I talked to this woman, she continued to smile and her eyes shone with merriment. It was so undeniably clear that her choice to be happy was sincere. She wasn't just saying words she thought others needed to hear so they wouldn't be upset about her move. She really meant it.

With the lesson I learned that day in mind, I'll work toward choosing happiness as much as I can for whatever years I have left; and if the time comes when I have to pack a shoebox, I'll try my best to do that with a smile.

Something I've learned in my seventy-plus years of living is that we don't have to be a hostage to our feelings. We can't help, or change, feelings. They're just there in all their glory, negative or positive. What we can do, however, is change the way we think and behave. As the wise man, Buddha, once said, "We are shaped by our thoughts. We become what we think."

So maybe the feelings can change as our thinking changes. Perhaps that was the secret to that woman's happiness, and maybe it can be a way for us, you and me, to choose to be happy. Maybe not all the time. That isn't realistic, and I'm sure in the privacy of her room that woman let the smile falter at times. But I'm equally sure that she gave herself a little shake after letting the sadness be there for a moment, then brought the smile to life again.

We can do that.

You can do that.

I can do that.

Not in the midst of that all-consuming grief when a major loss has first hit, but, as that heartache starts to slip away, maybe we can help it move along by our conscious decisions.

NOTE FROM THE AUTHOR

Thank you so much for taking the time to read my book. I do hope that you have found something enjoyable and helpful by reading all the stories and the little tidbits of wisdom I've included; and I'd be honored if you would consider leaving a review on Amazon. Those reviews do help an author so much.

Thank you,
Maryann

ABOUT THE AUTHOR

Maryann Miller is an award-winning author of numerous books, screenplays, and stage plays. She started her professional career as a journalist, writing columns, feature stories, and short fiction for regional and national publications. As a Public Relations consultant, she designed and wrote brochures, annual reports, and marketing material for a large financial institution.

Now she writes primarily mysteries, including the critically acclaimed *Seasons Mystery Series* that features two women homicide detectives. Think "Lethal Weapon" set in Dallas with female leads. The first two books in the series, *Open Season* and *Stalking Season* received starred reviews from Publisher's Weekly, Kirkus, and Library Journal. *Stalking Season* was chosen for the John E. Weaver Excellence in Reading award for Police Procedural Mysteries. Her mystery, *Double-take*, was honored as the Best Mystery for 2015 by the Texas Association of Authors.

A recent release, *Evelyn Evolving*, a story of real life debuted as a number one best-seller at Amazon when it was published by Next Chapter Publishing. It is the story of her mother's life, so naturally, very dear to her heart.

Miller no longer works as a chaplain, after having spent more than thirty years as a hospital minister, first as a volunteer, then in paid positions. For eight years she worked at Alegent Health in Omaha, NE, which is now CHI Immanuel, as well as Methodist Hospital. The departments she specialized in were oncology, med/surg, ICU, ER, and rehab. For three of those eight years, she ran two Grief Support Groups that met weekly.

After moving back to TX, she was a volunteer for Cypress Basin Hospice for three years

FOLLOW MARYANN MILLER:

maryannwrites.com

TWITTER - @maryannwrites

In addition to writing a personal blog, she's a contributor to The Blood-Red Pencil blog on writing and editing.